Food Combining

FOOD COMBINING FOR DYNAMIC ENERGY, WEIGHT LOSS, AND VITALITY AT ANY AGE

Tim Spong
and
Vicki Peterson

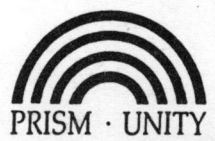

PRISM · UNITY

Published in Great Britain 1993 by
PRISM PRESS
2 South Street
Bridport
Dorset DT6 3NQ

Originally published in Australia by
SALLY MILNER PUBLISHING
558 Darling Street
Rozelle NSW 2039

ISBN 1 85327 079 2

© Write-On Publishing Pty Ltd, 1993
© recipes Tim Spong, 1993

All rights reserved. No part of this publication may be reproduced, stored in a retrieval system, or transmitted, in any form or by any means, electronic, mechanical, photocopying, recording or otherwise, without the prior permission of the publishers.

Printed by The Guernsey Press Ltd, The Channel Islands.

Cover:
Still Life 1926
Margaret Preston
Oil on canvas
50.8 x 56.0 cm
Bequest of Adrian Feint 1972
Collection: Art Gallery of New South Wales

Acknowledgements

Tim Spong
I would like to express my genuine thanks for the very real assistance given to me by the following people in preparing this book and reviewing the manuscript. The guidance and support from Eleanor Parker proved to be invaluable due to her background as a dietitian and her extensive knowledge of the Hopewood Health Care programme. Two of the finest Natural Therapists I have met, Greg Mathieson and Peter Ray, also played a significant role particularly with the knowledge I have aquired over the years about cleansing, FOOD COMBINING and Natural Health. Finally and perhaps most importantly, I would like to acknowledge one of the greatest and most profound learning experiences of my life, namely working at the Hopewood Health Centre at Wallacia, in particular the role played by the Chairman of the private charity that controls Hopewood, Mrs Madge Cockburn. Her genuine caring about the health of all people, her wisdom, knowledge of Natural Health and personal dedication to a healthy lifestyle, has had perhaps the greatest impact on my own development. Her balance as a person and her excellent health is an inspiration to all who have met her.

Vicki Peterson
Many individuals have contributed their inspiration and expert knowledge to this book.

I would like to sincerely thank the following: Dr Peter Theiss and his wife Barbara; Professor N. Shaternikov; Professor Jeremiah Stanning; Dr Abram Hoffer; Dr Mark Donohoe; Dr Gordon Latto; Dr David Lewis; Dr K. M. Shahani; Natasha Treven; Hans Wagner; Tim Ashton-Jennings.

Much of the original research for the book has been based on personal interviews or correspondence with these people.

Contents

	Acknowledgements	3
1	Time for a Change	7
2	Understanding the Food Groups	18
3	Understanding Digestion	28
4	Food Combining Charted	35
5	Say Goodbye to Bad Habits	39
6	Maintaining the Acid-Alkaline Balance	44
7	When and How Much to Eat	51
8	Detoxification	57
9	Losing Weight	65
10	The Need to be Active	69
11	Water—Beware!	73
12	Bountiful Bioflora	82
13	Yoghurt—Milk of Eternal Life	86
14	Green Power—the Power of Juice	90
15	Food Can Cure	97
16	Case Histories from Hopewood	108
17	What is a Healthy Lifestyle	113
18	Two Week Meal Planner	120
19	Recipes for Food Combining	127
20	Natural Foods—Their Nutritional Value and Combinations	168

Index to Recipes
Bibliography

1
Time for a Change

I have come to believe that eating food in harmonious combinations is one of the single greatest improvements you can make in your life. Let me also add that the changes you need to make in order to practise FOOD COMBINING are really very simple and easy to incorporate into your current lifestyle.

And the benefits are truly remarkable! That is the bonus you give yourself when you start taking responsibility for your own health and wellbeing.

Perhaps the recommendations I make in this book go against the grain of some of your existing eating habits.

We learn to eat when young and it quickly becomes a habit. Jam on bread, cheese or tomato sandwiches, ham on toast, sausage rolls—these are all delightful childhood snacks.

Breaking the eating habits of years is seldom accomplished overnight. It takes time to re-educate the palate and practise thinking about foods we have come to take for granted.

Examples of changing habits abound. What about those who have given up eating salt. At first they complain they can't taste food like tomatoes. But is it actually the food they can't taste? No, it's the salt! After a while their taste buds adjust and they begin to experience the wonderful taste of natural tomatoes. When salt is reintroduced by accident, they are the first to notice how *strong* it suddenly is on their palate.

It's the same with sugar. Many people have cut down or eliminated sugar in hot beverages such as tea and coffee. At first the weaning process off sugar is difficult and the drink tastes unpleasant, but in time sugar tastes sickly sweet and unpleasant when reintroduced, even in small amounts.

The fact that you are reading this book means that you are prepared to examine your eating habits. No doubt, you'll slip up at first, but don't be hard on yourself. If you get indigestion, or you feel off colour and your conscience nags you that you have eaten the wrong combinations of food, whatever you do don't feel guilty. It's what we do 95 per cent of the time that counts, not the 5 per cent. That's a forgiveable slip up the body can handle while you get used to FOOD COMBINING. Note your mistake and move on. Ask the family to follow FOOD COMBINING principles with you. This way you have everyone checking on the ingredients and discussing the different compatible foods. It begins as a game which gets easier the more you play it.

Ask the family for feedback. Check which meals seem easier to digest than others. After a week or two of FOOD COMBINING note how much more energy you all have.

Focus on the end result,—good health. That will help keep you on the right track.

Let me whet your appetite with a list of the major improvements you can expect.

- Your energy will increase in leaps and bounds.

- Digestive problems, indigestion and flatulence will diminish.

- You will look and feel younger.

- Your immune system will gradually strengthen.

- Losing weight will become easier. You can say goodbye to dieting, hunger and misery.

- You will begin to feel mentally brighter and more cheerful.

Now it is quite fair that you ask how the practice of eating certain foods at the same time can bring about such drastic change.

The great Japanese scientist, Dr Yoshihide Hagiwara states categorically: 'Our bodies can only function normally when the digestive and entire enzyme system is allowed to function normally.'

And that is what FOOD COMBINING will do. It will allow the digestive and enzyme system to function normally.

There are only a few separate points which describe FOOD COMBINING briefly, and these are set out below. I will expand upon each of them in later chapters, but these are the foundations.

1 First, different foods need quite different digestive enzymes to be digested properly. Foods such as nuts, cheese, and all meats (commonly classed as proteins) need an 'acid environment' in order to digest properly. On the other hand, foods such as potatoes, rice, bread and cake (commonly classed as starch foods) need a predominantly 'alkaline environment' in which to digest. Eat them both at the same time and you create a digestive battlefield right from the first mouthful.

For example, when you eat protein (meat) with starch (potato) at the same time, your system pours various enzymes into action, diluting and weakening the action of each other. When you eat protein (meat) with fat (oil, butter, etc) the fat slows down the movement of food through the stomach and intestines, thereby lengthening the digestive time.

2 Second, fluid should not be taken with meals. A leading British dietary expert, Dr Gordon Latto, has been teaching for years that liquids drunk during meals dilute the digestive enzymes, further slowing down the digestive procedure. Under our guidelines you should drink at least half an hour before or some hours after meals, and avoid all extremes of temperatures in food and drinks because cold temperatures retard or slow down enzyme action and very hot, or boiling, will destroy or stop it altogether.

3 Alkaline foods (i.e. vegetables, most fruits) should make up the largest proportion of all the food you eat. We suggest that three quarters of our food intake should be alkaline (basically vegetables, fruit) and one quarter acid (basically proteins) — (see chapter 7).

4 Fruit should be eaten alone or with compatible foods. Sweet fruits combine with starch foods. Acid fruits combine with protein foods.

5 Milk should really be left for infants. It is more difficult to digest after our permanent teeth are formed. It may be taken as cheese, butter or yoghurt, which are pre-curdled, or partly-digested (see chapter 13).

We also recommend that you 'detoxify' or cleanse your body before you start a change of diet. This will clear away a build-up of toxins already in your system and give you a head start (see chapter 8).

Results of Improper Food Combining

Improper FOOD COMBINING leads to bad digestion and a body battling bad digestion, will, in the long term suffer. That's because good digestion and proper, easy absorption of food is at the very core of good health.

Let's consider what happens when conflicting foods come together inside you. Obviously, one type of food has to wait for the other to digest. This means a meal consisting of, say, proteins (fish), starch (potato) and fats (cooking oil) can remain in the stomach six to seven hours before the stomach finally empties itself ready for another meal.

But who waits for seven hours to eat again? Most of us eat by the clock and, hungry or not, we tip another incompatible meal right on top of our already overloaded digestive system.

The result?

The food which is partly digested or is waiting to be digested begins to putrify. The body signals its distress with flatulence or stomach pain and, because it's working overtime, energy for other things is diverted to the digestive process.

It takes a lot of energy to digest food. You can remember how sleepy and lethargic you feel after Christmas or other festive meals. Even a snack 'eaten on the run' takes a surprising amount of energy to digest.

Improperly combined food takes up much, much more energy. The distinguished American, Dr Herbert M. Shelton, who researched FOOD COMBINING for over 40 years, estimated that it needs as much energy to digest a poor combination of food as it does to run nearly a kilometre at your fastest speed.

If poorly combined food is eaten on a regular basis, then the result is regular indigestion, bloating, lethargy, poor assimilation of food which leads to fatty, toxic-laden deposits in the body, or, to put it simply, weight gain. Coupled with this, the body often becomes chemically-imbalanced.

In some people, poorly combined food and irregular body chemistry can lead to constant hunger and no feelings of satisfaction, no matter how much they have eaten. This is what the Nobel Prize winner, Dr Roger Williams, calls 'a state of cellular malnutrition'. It occurs because your body cannot properly assimilate all the essential vitamins and minerals.

Similarly, frontline researchers, such as Dr Roy Walford, have recently discovered how vitally important properly functioning digestive enzymes are in regulating hormone function and the immune system itself, especially as our bodies age.

The Founder of Food Combining

We have been practising FOOD COMBINING at Hopewood Health Centre for 30 years, introducing it to literally thousands of people, with enormous success. However, we certainly did not devise the system.

It is a system of eating which was first introduced by Dr William Howard Hay, an American who was born in Hartstown, Pennsylvania in 1866.

A graduate of the University of New York, Hay practised medicine for sixteen years and by the end of that time his health had seriously deteriorated. He had developed Bright's disease, high blood pressure and, finally, a dilated heart. Naturally, he thought his career was over. Even his doctors advised him to 'put his affairs in order'.

Hay, believing he had nothing to lose, decided to treat himself. He began 'eating fundamentally' as he described it, foods in their natural unprocessed state, and in moderate quantities. To the amazement of his doctors, his symptoms gradually disappeared and, by the end of twelve weeks, he felt fit and strong. He'd lost over twenty-three kilograms and could run long distances without distress.

He wrote in the medical journals of the day that medicine was on the wrong track, fussing with the end results of illness, instead of removing the causes. He had proved, on himself, that the body could cure itself, given the right diet. For the next four years he spent his time treating his patients through diet to prove or disprove his theory that 'we are what we eat'.

Over the subsequent years, until his death in 1940, he developed a system of eating he called FOOD COMBINING. He taught his patients that there were four main causes of the condition he called autointoxication (toxaemia, self-poisoning), which lowered the body's vital alkaline reserve, creating the wrong chemical conditions for proper digestion.

These were:
1 Too much consumption of meat.
2 Overuse of refined carbohydrates (white flour products) and refined sugar.
3 A dismal mix of food which caused indigestion.
4 Constipation.

He argued that although young people built up a tolerance to incompatible mixtures, just as people build up a tolerance to alcohol, they did so at the price of lost vitality and, as they grew older, chronic bad health.

Hay was attacked for teaching that prevention was better than treatment and was written off as a quack. Practitioners at the time were supporters of 'the germ theory of disease' and enthusiastic about the new wonder drugs. They rejected nutritional therapy, scorning its simplicity. However, when Dr Hay was seventy-four his work was finally recognised as worthwhile, as doctors began to appreciate the link between nutrition and good health.

The American, Dr Shelton, mentioned earlier, was a Hay disciple who founded the Natural Hygiene Society in the United States in 1949, to educate the general public in a natural, healthy lifestyle based on the twin studies of biology and physiology.

Shelton taught thousands of people basic FOOD COMBINING principles because he believed that good health depended on the digestive tract breaking down the food properly, both physically and chemically, without creating any excess toxic substances.

He wrote 'the digestion of food requires more energy than any other single bodily activity. The aim therefore, is to put as little stress on the digestive tract as possible during digestion.

'Each food has its own requirements. FOOD COMBINING simply attempts to combine, at the same meal, foods with similar digestive requirements and foods which harmonise with each other during digestion.'

Food Combining is Commonsense

By now I hope this simple concept which promotes good digestion, is ringing a bell of truth. For me FOOD COMBINING is, quite simply, common sense.

What is so exciting about this concept is that you don't have to understand or believe it from a theoretical point of view. Just experiencing the wonderful lifts in vitality and a sense of wellbeing will convert you to the principles of FOOD COMBINING.

The resulting improvement in digestion and the absorption of essential nutrients, is undoubtedly the key to a remarkable improvement in health and vitality.

Don't take my word. Try it out yourself. But let me give you this assurance. I have seen jaded, overweight and ill men, women and teenagers transform their health and revitalise their lives on this system, starting with a period of cleansing and then going on to proper FOOD COMBINING with abundant fruits and vegetables and juices.

Hopewood Health Centre has received glowing testimonials from our guests and the founders of the Centre also raised 85 children to adulthood who had been placed in their care before the Centre was established. The children set world records in dental hygiene and health care.

When you increase your daily intake of foods such as fresh fruit and vegetables and when you practise proper FOOD COMBINING so that digestion is easy and efficient, your system begins to work in a harmonious way. You will not only feel more energetic, but you will begin to feel physically and mentally renewed.

Furthermore, it has been recorded that the number one and number two killer diseases in the United States of America (and Australia follows America's lead) are heart disease and cancer respectively. In their book *Fit for Life*, Marilyn and Harvey Diamond write that the latest information released by the scientific community, is an increase of fruit and vegetables in a person's diet can decrease the incidence of both these killers.

In 1982 doctors at the National Cancer Institute in America said: 'Changing the way we eat could offer some protection against cancer. The first guideline is to reduce fat. The second is to increase the intake of fruit and vegetables.' It is little wonder that diet is now one of the major areas of research into cancer prevention.

By FOOD COMBINING, undergoing regular cleansing and making sure that alkaline foods in your meals are well in excess of the acid intake, you will not only lose weight, and keep that weight off, you will reduce your risk of premature heart disease and cancer.

It's only habit which makes us eat heavy meals in the

morning and at night. Habit again which causes us to mix proteins and starches. And it's habit that makes us eat fruit after meals and snack between meals. It is vital that you start to accept new habits, for your health's sake. And the way to do that is to crowd out old habits with new habits. You don't have to change your way of eating overnight. Do it gradually and seek help. Learn how to FOOD COMBINE correctly.

You only have one body. If you abuse it then it will falter and become diseased. The key to long term good health lies with the concept of prevention. The real strength of natural health is built on this foundation. This doesn't mean that you are a lost cause if you already have a health problem. Focus on preventing the problem from becoming worse while you seek to cure it.

Love your body. Show your appreciation by being kind to it. Give it a chance to function at its highest level, unburdened by toxic waste and unwanted fat.

When you start to experience good health and vitality you will come to appreciate what a fine instrument you live within and thus learn to be proud of your body. Enjoy yourself and watch a slender healthy you emerge.

Take pride in never getting sick and knowing that your immune system is strengthened by the way you choose to live your life. Mentally your spirits will lift if your body is feeling good. It's a two way street. Mind and body are interlinked as I have already said. You can't feel good if you aren't caring for the house in which your mind resides.

Don't let anyone tell you you can't have fun and enjoy yourself while you eat well. These remarks are designed to make the other person feel safe while he or she watches you make a stand for your health's sake. It is a funny thing about human nature, but we like to run with the herd, even when the herd is being destructive. It takes courage to stand up amongst the herd and say: 'I choose to be with you, but I wish to be different.'

Being different pays health dividends. In the long term you will stay younger, fitter and have a quality of life that far surpasses those who foolishly criticise you for being 'a goody "food" shoes'.

By example we teach. Make yourself a teacher and don't be afraid to go against the tide now—for the tide is turning, believe me. I predict that regular detoxification programmes, FOOD COMBINING and fitness programmes will be recognised by everyone as the only way to live by the turn of this century.

2
Understanding the Food Groups

First, let's look at what is meant by good food. Many people believe all food is good for you, provided it is not stale, or poisoned with chemicals during its production.

Food which is detrimental to our health
What they overlook is that food can be damaging as well as nourishing. At the beginning of this century, health researchers such as Dr William Howard Hay and Dr Alexis Carrol defined food as being 'substances which convert into blood, flesh, bone and nerve.' Anything that didn't become living structure was termed poisonous.

These two men found there were some food particles which could pass through the digestive tract and which were neutral provided they didn't enter the bloodstream. These ranged in toxicity from nearly neutral to virulent enough to cause illness. For instance, tobacco is a plant which contains vitamins, minerals and proteins, like other plants, but it also contains poisons that make it totally unfit for us to eat. There are many other substances like this that have food value. Belladonna is poisonous to humans, but excellent food for rabbits because the rabbit has enzymes that digest the Belladonna poisons.

Wine, beer, brandy, whiskey, ale, rum and vodka are all drinks that are can be thought of as food, because they contain substances such as carbohydrates and small amounts of minerals and vitamins. Yet alcohol, especially when it is drunk in excess, is a poison which compromises digestion, so the goodness is not readily available to our bodies.

Sodium and chloride, as well as mineral salts, are in all food, yet salt in excess can be detrimental. We season our food with table salt and other strong condiments which only upset our digestion and may cause long-term side effects.

At Hopewood Health Centre, one of the first things we do is encourage people to 'taste' and enjoy their meals without salt, pepper and other strongly flavoured boosters. When required, we only use totally natural seasoning and fresh herbs. At first, people who are used to highly seasoned food say they can't taste the food without the seasoning. But after their taste buds adjust they start to experience the real taste of food again.

Foods which nourish
The foods which nourish us best consist of proteins, carbohydrates, fats, mineral salts and vitamins. None of these food groups taken alone can sustain life for long. In fact no single type of food is capable of maintaining healthy life indefinitely, because no animal, humans included, can live a long healthy life on mono-diets.

We need a variety of food to keep us truly healthy, to give us a balance of all the food groups on a daily basis.

Let's look at these important food groups:

Protein Food
Protein is the basic structure of every living cell and vital to good health. It is considered the 'building blocks' of life and is composed of valuable amino acids. Our bodies can't store protein, so we need it in our diet on a daily basis.

The following foods have a high protein composition:

SEEDS (pumpkin, sunflower, sesame, linseed, etc)
NUTS (hazelnuts, almonds, cashews, etc)
DAIRY PRODUCTS (yoghurt, cheese)
SOY BEANS
EGGS
PEANUTS
FLESH FOODS (fish, shellfish, poultry, red meat)
TOFU
TEMPEH

Carbohydrate Food (Starches and Sugars)

The most prolific nutrients in nature, carbohydrates should constitute the bulk of our diet. That's because our bodies use it as fuel which is burnt off when we are active. Unused 'fuel' is stored in the fatty tissue as reserves.

Carbohydrates have a high percentage of either starch or sugar in their composition, which is why I have broken them into several categories.

The high starchy foods are:

ALL GRAINS (rice, wheat, oats, rye, barley, buckwheat, millet)
DRY BEANS AND PULSES (adzuki beans, chickpeas, mung beans, lentils, butter beans, etc)
POTATOES (all kinds)
PEAS
CORN
SWEET POTATOES
PUMPKINS
PARSNIPS
ARTICHOKES

CHESTNUTS
YAM
TARO.

The syrups and sugared foods are:
MAPLE SYRUP, MOLASSES, HONEY, JAM, GOLDEN SYRUP, TREACLE, etc.

Fruits

These are the 'energy boosters', for fruit sugar is the easiest of all foods to digest. It provides a quick energy source, as well as vital minerals and vitamins which the body needs to maintain healthy bones, tissues and nerves.

Fruits are divided into several sub-categories.

The sweet fruits are:
RIPE BANANA
DATE
DRIED FIGS
RAISIN AND OTHER DRIED FRUITS
PERSIMMON
MANGOSTEEN
MANGO
other tropical fruits such as CUSTARD APPLES.

The neutral fruit that goes equally well with any type of starch or protein food is:
PAWPAW

The acid fruits are:
BLACKBERRY
GRAPEFRUIT
KIWIFRUIT
LEMON

ORANGE
PINEAPPLE
PLUM
RASPBERRIES
STRAWBERRIES, etc.

Note that the TOMATO, commonly thought of as a vegetable, is an *acid fruit*.

The sub-acid fruits are:
APPLE
APRICOT
BLACKCURRANTS
FRESH FIGS
GRAPES
NECTARINE
PEACH
PEAR
CHERRIES, etc.

Melons
Because of their high sugar and water content, they digest quickly and so these sweet fruits are better eaten on their own. They are:
WATER MELON
SUGAR MELON
HONEY DEW
ROCK MELON.

Fats and Oils
These contain valuable nutrients and are essential in everyone's diet in moderate amounts. Natural fats and oils are composed of a mixture of saturated fatty acids, mono-unsaturated fatty acids and polyunsaturated fatty acids.

The foods which have considerable quantities of fat in their composition are:
VEGETABLE OILS (olive oil, soy oil, sunflower seed oil, sesame oil, corn oil)
MILK FAT (butter, cream, full cream cheese)
MEAT FATS (ie lard, dripping, suet)
MARGARINE
COCONUT.

Non-Starchy and Green Vegetables
These are valuable to health because of their vitamins and mineral salts. They are, however, low in proteins, carbohydrates and fats, so they need to be eaten with foods from the other groups.

They are:
LETTUCE
CELERY
ENDIVE
CHICORY
CABBAGE
CAULIFLOWER
BROCCOLI
BRUSSELS SPROUTS
SPINACH
OKRA
CHINESE CABBAGE
CHIVE
TURNIP
EGGPLANT
GREEN BEANS
CUCUMBER
SORREL
PARSLEY

RHUBARB
WATER CRESS
ONIONS
SCALLIONS
LEEKS
GARLIC
ZUCCHINI
BAMBOO SPROUTS
SUMMER SQUASH
ASPARAGUS
RADISH
CAPSICUM.

Eat a Big Variety

Food classifications like those given on the previous pages are guidelines. They cannot be rigid groupings because nature produces no pure proteins, carbohyrates, fats, minerals and vitamins. Most foods contain a mixture, although most naturally occurring food is strong in only one of the major food groups listed above. For example, most food that contains a considerable amount of protein does not contain a large amount of carbohydrate.

That is why we must try to eat as big a *variety* of natural foods as possible, to ensure we get adequate amounts of vitamins, minerals, energy 'fuel' and amino acids. However, as you are starting to discover, this variety should be taken over the day, not in any one meal.

Vitamins

Vitamins exist in all foods in minute quantities. The body uses them to help it assimilate or synegistically absorb the various nutrients. We, in our modern laboratories, have managed to chemically duplicate these vitamins which are sold as food supplements to assist our nutritionally depleted, processed, refined and artificially flavoured food.

What we have to realise is that the body needs a varied diet of fruit, nuts, vegetables and other natural foods if it is to work efficiently. Refined and processed foods, boosted by artificial vitamins can never duplicate nature's beautifully balanced combinations.

Nutrients often work together, in combination with other elements. These are superbly balanced in fresh whole foods. Thus taking artificial supplements over long periods of time, can cause deficiencies, or more commonly toxic reactions.

Furthermore, the chemicals added to processed foods for colour, flavour, etc can contribute to a whole host of other problems. Some people have quite violent reactions to these additives.

And though vitamins are in everything that grows, they are easily destroyed when extracted from their natural sources.

Alfalfa is a rich source of vitamin C, but when it is cut and left to dry in the field, it loses 70 per cent of its vitamin C content in one day. When it is dried, powdered and pressed into tablets, there is no vitamin C left. So you can see that a fresh alfalfa salad is much better for you than an alfalfa tablet.

Nourishment is paramount

As Dr David Phillips notes in his book *New Dimensions in Health—from Soil to Psyche*, the two basic purposes of food are to nourish the body and stimulate the senses.

Think of how wonderful freshly-baked white bread is when it's just left the oven, and how the mouth waters for a tantalising strawberry cream sponge. Both these temptations lack nourishment, but are extremely satisfying to the senses.

What we have to realise is that nourishment is much too important to ignore, as we weigh up the white bread against the natural grain brown bread and a bowl of freshly picked strawberries against the pureed strawberry cream sponge.

Today, it seems almost impossible to fully satisfy the need for nourishment and the need to stimulate while science continues to tinker with the flavour, colour and texture of food. At the moment it seems the stimulation of the senses takes priority over nourishment. And confused, the body craves for the foods which poison it, rejecting the foods which nourish.

Already several generations of children are suffering from nutritional imbalance and lifestyle disorders, rather than give up the tasty foods that tempt them. The popularity of fast foods such as hamburgers, pizzas, fried chicken pieces, fish in batter with chips, chicko rolls, sausage rolls, pies, curried puffs and a host of others are proof enough that we are already hooked by our tyrannical taste buds.

The only way to combat this artificially-created addiction, is to make the decision to take responsibility for every morsel of food we put in our mouths. If the end result is good health and a happy mental attitude, then the price is small to pay.

To get started, begin by evaluating the nourishment of every edible item you buy. Remember, as I said in the beginning of this chapter, food is defined as that which converts to living tissue.

Be aware that modern science is tampering with nature and the result is food which is often depleted nutritionally and which can cause a whole host of health problems because of the chemicals which are used in the processing.

It's your choice to replace part or all of this food with a food programme that emphasises plenty of fresh vegetables and fruit, nuts and seeds, limited amounts of cereals, meat and dairy products. But remember, appropriately combined vegetarian sources of protein are necessary if you choose to eliminate flesh foods from your diet.

Don't take my word for it. Try it out for yourself. See what works for you and what you feel comfortable with. For a month test out a food programme of whole unprocessed foods, instead of one consisting of highly processed food, and see how you look and feel.

The body is a remarkable mechanism. It responds and adapts and heals—and it has a language you can easily understand if you start tuning in.

3
Understanding Digestion

To properly understand FOOD COMBINING, you must first understand how your digestive system works and how it deals with the food you eat.

The body is highly adaptable and can deal with all food very efficiently. It can suit its fluids and enzymes to the character of the food that is eaten, and to the complexity of the food. What it finds difficult and stressful is adapting the juices to the *variety* of food eaten at once.

For example, digestion begins in the mouth with the salivary enzyme Ptyalin. The optimum pH factor in the mouth is 6.7 which is neutral to slightly acid. (The pH factor is the measure of acidity.) A pH of 7 is neutral, a pH of less than 7 is acid and greater than 7 is alkaline (see chapter 7).

The gastric enzyme Pepsin in the stomach initiates protein digestion and is active only in an acid medium (i.e. less than 7). Alkalines such as soda and antacids destroy the proper medium for this activity.

Very simply, it is because these two very important enzymes need very different environments, that we need to consider the make-up of the various foods we eat together.

Let us look in more detail at the digestive process of the main food groups.

Proteins
Gastric juice, the main enzyme of which is Pepsin, ranging in strength from neutral to strongly acid, depending on the

character of the food, breaks the proteins into simple units called Peptides. Other enzymes in the small intestine break the Peptides into amino acids which are carried into the blood stream as nutrients for the cells.

Pepsin can only act in an acid medium through the secretion of hydrochloric acid, which is produced by the gastric glands in the stomach.

Proteins such as nuts and seeds, or various kinds of cheese, digest well together, even though they require different digestive sequences. For example, plant proteins require early low acidity of pH 5.5. Later the acidity rises to pH 4.0.

Cheese commences at pH 3.5, later reaching pH 3.0, and eggs begin at pH 3.5 later reaching pH 2.0.

(In humans a pH of 1.6 is the most acidic level possible.)

Meat is digested by meat eating animals at a gastric pH of 1.0 which is stronger than the maximum human level. Therefore the human stomach holds a pH of 2.0 for many hours in order to break down meat protein.

Because of the different levels of acid concentration, and different secretion times for each type of protein, the following simple rules ensure efficient protein digestion.

RULE 1 *Avoid eating too many different proteins (e.g. meat, nuts, cheese and eggs) at the same meal. Free fats such as butter, fried foods, etc coat the gastric mucosa, preventing the stomach from secreting gastric juice and thus delaying protein digestion.*

RULE 2 *Eat fats and proteins at separate meals. If they must be eaten together, then eat a raw green vegetable salad to help counteract the inhibiting effect of the fats.*

Sugars such as sweet fruits, honey, etc undergo little digestion in the mouth or stomach, passing through the digestive process in 15 to 20 minutes. If they are held up by protein in the stomach, they ferment and cause intestinal gas.

RULE 3 *When eating proteins the best combination is with green vegetables. However, acid fruits go well with low strength proteins such as cottage cheese, cream cheese, yoghurt, nuts and seeds.*

Carbohydrates

All carbohydrates consist of starches and sugars or combinations of sugars which are called saccharides. Single sugar units, such as glucose and fructose, are called monosaccharides. A saccharide containing two sugars is called a disaccharide, e.g. sucrose or cane sugar. Foods which contain many sugars are called polysaccharides, e.g. starch. Therefore starch is simply a large number of sugars combined together.

Grains are high in starches, while fruits are high in sugar. Another type of carbohydrate is cellulose (fibre) which is not absorbed into the bloodstream, but provides important roughage.

Unlike protein or fat, carbohydrates leave no complex waste products when they are burnt off for energy, so they do not put any pressure on the eliminative organs such as the kidneys and liver.

Foods which must be most abundant in a good diet are carbohydrates such as fruits, salads, vegetables and grains. They are essential for energy, but most people eat far too much refined carbohydrates e.g. bread, candy bars etc.

Starches

Digestion of starch starts in the mouth with saliva containing the enzyme Ptyalin which acts best in a neutral or mildly alkaline environment. This enzyme breaks down starch to Maltose, a sugar which is then acted upon by the Maltose enzyme in the small intestine, converting it to simple sugar.

The pancreas secretes the enzyme Amylase which acts on the starch in the small intestine as does Ptyalin in the mouth.

Thus any starch missed by Ptyalin (if food is bolted and not chewed properly) can be dealt with further on in the digestive process.

Two rules for starch digestion are:

RULE 1 *Avoid eating starch and protein foods at the same meal. Starch digestion stops in the acid stomach environment so starch foods pass fairly quickly through the stomach. Protein foods, on the other hand, undergo digestion in the stomach and are held in the stomach for a longer period of time. Eating the two together creates a 'compromise' in the digestion of starches and proteins. For example, bread rolls with fish or chicken, potatoes and meat are poor combinations.*

RULE 2 *Avoid eating starch and acid foods together. Remember, the starch digesting enzyme, Ptyalin, is unactivated in the presence of acids. Say goodbye to tomato sandwiches and tomato sauce on pasta. It is always best to eat vegetables with starchy foods.*

Fruit

Fresh fruits are easily digested because they have low protein, low fat, high water content, are high in enzymes and vitamins and are able to pass quickly through the stomach. They also have low starch levels so they are quickly absorbed through the small intestine.

It is because of their speedy digestion, that fruits must not be eaten too soon after meals, as they sit on top of that meal and ferment.

Three rules to remember when eating fruit are:

RULE 1   *Fruits are best eaten at a fruit meal alone. But they can be tolerated when eaten with other foods that require similar digestive situations e.g. sweet fruits combine acceptably with carbohydrates and acid fruits can be eaten with protein-rich foods.*

RULE 2   *Sweet starchy fruits such as bananas are best not eaten with acid fruits such as oranges, plums, etc. Because acid fruits don't ferment it is alright to combine these with small amounts of protein such as nuts or fresh cheese or yoghurt.*

RULE 3   *Melons, because of their high water and sugar content, are best eaten alone.*

Fat

Fats and oils are common lipids called triglycerides. Each triglyceride contains three fatty acids. During digestion the fatty acids are split off the triglycerides and absorbed separately. Thus we eat fats, but absorb fatty acids.

Cholesterol is a type of lipid and is often confused with fats and oils. It is an important substance found in the cell membrane of every cell in the body. It is also the basis for several hormones. Manufactured by the liver for use throughout the body, cholesterol plays no part in the plant kingdom and is therefore not found in any plant food.

It is only found in red meats, white meats, shellfish and fish, dairy products and eggs. Because saturated fats and cholesterol are usually found together in animal foods, they are often confused with each other.

Plant foods may also have fats. The most popular are avocadoes and olives and you can eat them in moderation.

Avocadoes and olives have a high oil content, the fatty acids of which help reduce cholesterol in people who are not overweight. However, if you are battling overweight, then despite their goodness, both these foods are best left off your food list until FOOD COMBINING has corrected your weight problem.

Milk

Milk is an alkaline substance and requires only a light concentration of gastric juice to digest it. However the protein in milk requires Rennin to coagulate the milk into curd, which the Pepsin is then able to break down.

While there is ample Rennin in an infant's stomach, this gradually disappears in adults, making proper digestion difficult. To compensate, the stomach secretes large quantities of mucus which turns the milk sour.

It is interesting that human milk passes through a baby's stomach in less than an hour, while cow's milk with three times the protein level, takes from one to two hours. If milk is taken with other proteins, the milk curds surround the other food, slowing down digestion, until the curds are broken down.

A rule to keep in mind when drinking milk is:

RULE 1 *Always drink milk alone. Adults are wise not to take any type of milk. Soft white cheeses, butter, yellow cheese and raw unsweetened yoghurt are the most acceptable dairy products for older children and adults.*

Now if you are beginning to feel that your whole enjoyment in food is being threatened by rigid rules, just remember the golden benefits of good digestion:

BUBBLING VITALITY

PERMANENT WEIGHT CONTROL

GOOD HEALTH *and*

FEELINGS OF HAPPINESS AND WELLBEING.

This is no idle promise, believe me. I have been FOOD COMBINING for years and I wake up each morning feeling really alive. I admit I found it a little difficult at first, but when you start slowly working with the guidelines, the whole process gets easier and easier.

Try eating this way for several months. See for yourself how rejuvenated and alive you feel.

4
Food Combining Charted

The following pages are designed for easy reference.

Each page is complete in itself and tells you one part of the FOOD COMBINING story.

There are 4 pages and each could be photocopied and carried with you for ease of reference.

Foods to be Avoided
Following is a list of acid-forming foods or substances which should be avoided or kept to a minimum:

meat	all drugs
fish	coffee
chicken	tea
cheese	vinegar
milk (except for babies)	alcohol
all flour-sugar products	

FOOD COMBINING is based on the concept that different enzymes digest different types of food. If you keep your food intake within certain groups you will digest and absorb meals much more easily and your body will utilise the vitamins and minerals in the food more efficiently.

Uncomplicated combinations of food can:
— eliminate digestive problems
— help control your weight
— prevent flatulence

Recommendations:
1. Do not eat concentrated proteins (cheese, nuts, meat, eggs, fish) with concentrated starches (cereals, bread, potatoes, biscuits, etc).
2. Green vegetables and salads, eggplant, carrots, avocadoes and mushrooms are classed as neutral foods and may be eaten with either starch or protein food.
3. Do not drink with meals, this dilutes the digestive juices and delays digestion.
4. If you have protein for lunch have starch for dinner or vice versa.
5. Do not eat acid fruit (oranges, pineapple, grapefruit, passionfruit, etc) with starchy foods (cereals, potatoes, etc).
6. Avoid eating sweet foods (raisins, dates, honey, bananas, etc) with acid fruits.
7. Whilst fats such as unsalted butter and cold pressed oils combine with either starch or protein food they should be used sparingly.
8. Melons are best eaten alone or at least 10 minutes before other foods because of their high fluid content and rapid digestion.

Basic Food Groups

Starches
potatoes
bread
rice
corn
bananas
biscuits/cake
cereals/grains
pumpkin
lentils
buckwheat

Proteins
cheese
yoghurt
nuts
seeds (sunflower and sesame)
nut butters
beans, e.g. soya, etc
chicken
fish
meat
eggs
coconut

Concentrated fats/oils
butter (unsalted)
oils (cold pressed)
cream
mayonnaise
olives
coconut

Acid fruits
grapefruit
oranges
pineapple
mandarins
lemons
tomatoes
kiwi fruit
strawberries
passionfruit

Sweet fruits
bananas
all dried fruits
persimmons
ripe mango
custard apples
sweet grapes
figs

Sub-acid fruits
apricots
plums
grapes
apples
pears
nectarines
peaches
berries
cherries
mango

Neutral fruits
avocados
paw paw

Vegetables
All vegetables and sprouts are neutral with the exception of potato, pumpkin, sweet potatoes, beetroot

Melons
eaten alone or prior to meal

FOOD COMBINING

Read down the first column and then across for the combination.

	Protein	Starch	Fats/Oils	Vegetables	Sweet Fruits	Sub-Acid Fruits	Acid Fruits
Protein	Yes	No	Yes*	Yes	No	Yes*	Yes
Starch	No	Yes	Yes*	Yes	Yes	Yes*	No
Fats/Oils	Yes*	Yes*	Yes*	Yes*	Yes*	Yes*	Yes*
Vegetables	Yes	Yes	Yes*	Yes	Yes	Yes	Yes
Sweet Fruits	No	Yes	Yes*	Yes	Yes	Yes	No
Sub-Acid Fruits	Yes*	Yes*	Yes*	Yes	Yes*	Yes	Yes
Acid Fruits	Yes	No	Yes*	Yes	No	Yes	Yes

*denotes combinations to be used only in moderation.

5
Say Goodbye to Bad Habits

Many dietitians disagree the FOOD COMBINING theory. They contend that most foods are digestible taken in combination with other foods, because all foods contain a number of different elements in the natural state (i.e. proteins, starches, fats, etc). But what is important to remember is that nature does *not* produce many foods which have more than one of these elements in a concentrated form. For example, a potato has both starch and protein, but the amount of protein is so insignificant compared to the starch that digestion is not disrupted.

At Hopewood, we have observed thousands of people on our FOOD COMBINING programme over the years and I can assure you that many of them report a lift in vitality, better digestion and loss of weight.

As any culinary student knows, cuisine is becoming an art form. Cook books abound with recipes which combine all sorts of ingredients in delectable and tantalising ways. But unfortunately these combinations can be unhealthy.

Perhaps the most damaging to digestion is the 'nouvelle cuisine' school which goes to imaginative lengths to mix meat with any number of incompatible sauces and trimmings. It may look exquisite, that small portion of chicken breast gently bathed in persimmon purée with grated lemon rind, finished off with a sprinkle of pine nuts, but how is the stomach meant to deal easily with such a rich combination of exotic ingredients.

For a start, as we have learnt in the previous chapters, sweet fruit is rich in natural sugar which quickly digests. It ferments in the digestive tract while it waits its turn, held up by the rich oily chicken and nuts. Are you really surprised when embarrassing flatulence occurs?

Let's look too, at the popular hamburger. The protein beef is dealt with by Pepsin, which is a strong acid enzyme in the stomach. When the starchy bun goes into the mouth, it is partly broken down by the Ptyalin enzyme in the saliva. Once in the stomach, the starch must sit and wait. The enzyme Ptyalin cannot continue to digest the starch as hydrochloric acid stops it, while the enzyme Pepsin breaks down the meat.

If a sugary milkshake follows the hamburger, which it often does, there is real trouble. The fatty milk not only dilutes the gastric juice, but also coats the gastric mucosa in the stomach and inhibits proper and efficient secretion of the digestive juices, further delaying digestion. (At Hopewood, milk is not even on the menu simply because it is considered unnecessary in an adult diet. We serve our natural muesli soaked in apple juice which not only tastes great, but also makes the cereal easier to digest.)

Alone, the hamburger meat is tasty and easily digested. With the bun it's heavy going and I don't mean just filling, but hard for the stomach to break down while it is dealing with the protein. The same applies to the ubiquitous pizza. The dough is starchy, the filling often protein— seafood or sausage meats. Even the vegetarian pizza causes problems because of the generous amount of cheese which binds the filling topside. Ideally you are better to eat the fillings and cheese by themselves and several hours later, once digestion is complete, chase it with the doughy base.

Another quick delicious dish with disharmonious components is the quiche. The doughy base fights with the protein in the eggs and ham. Even the vegetable quiche doesn't escape the poor combination of protein (egg) and starch (crust).

But the ultimate disastrous combination—even worse than protein and starch—is protein and fat. That favourite fast food, fried fish in batter and chips, tops the lists of bad combinations. You have starch, protein and fat together and as such it takes simply hours to digest. Your system is flat out disposing of this badly combined meal.

If you really want your digestion to work in peak form, then you have to consider foods like these you take for granted. Hamburgers, cheese and ham sandwiches, fish and chips, quiche, pizzas, meat pies, sausage rolls, all lack harmonious elements for proper digestion. They mix starch and protein, protein and fat. In FOOD COMBINING terms, this couldn't be worse, especially when you understand how digestion works and what happens when various foods are present at once in the stomach.

On the next page is a simple list of *Badly Combined Foods* and some *Excellent Alternatives.*

Keep a list like this for yourself and add to it as you learn more.

Badly Combined Foods	**Alternatives**
Quiche	leave off base
Pizza	vegetable only with no cheese
Pasta with meat or tomato sauce	pasta with vegetable sauce (e.g. spinach)

Meat pies	vegetable pastie
Hamburgers	without the bun
Curried puffs	vegetable curried puffs
Fried chicken and chips	grilled or roast chicken with salad or non starchy vegetables
Fish and chips	without batter, no chips, with salad
Meat and salad sandwich	salad sandwich only (no tomato)
Cheese sandwich	cheese and egg garden salad
Cereal with milk	cereal with fruit juice
Baked beans on toast	soya beans in tomato sauce

Take heart. FOOD COMBINING is not difficult. It just means adjusting your eating habits. If you want to eat quiche, then make it without the base. Egg, cheese and meat and most vegetables all go hand-in-hand.

Leave the cheese off the vegetable pizza. Most vegetables and starches love one another. (See the food list in Chapter 19).

Meat pies can't be revamped, but hamburgers can be eaten without the bun. Renamed 'the Clayton's burger' the meat can be loaded with onions and fresh salad and it will be easily dealt with by the body.

What about curried puffs and fried chicken. Well, chicken eaten alone or with a delicious fresh salad makes a wonderful compatible meal and vegetable curried puffs make nicer companions than meat filled puffs.

I know you will groan, but fish minus batter and chips, but with a salad companion only, is far better for you. If you simply love chips, eat them alone or with other salad and starch combinations.

Ideal Meal Plan

The ideal meal plan when FOOD COMBINING, in order to get the widest variety of foods and to get a balance of all the food groups, is:

- One protein meal per day. This could be grilled steak, accompanied by cooked vegetables, or cold chicken served with raw vegetable salad, or, for the vegetarian, soybean casserole with a variety of salad vegetables.

- One starch meal per day. This could be wholewheat bread and butter with salad filling or a choice of dates, raisins, figs and bananas.

- One meal per day which consists wholly of fresh, ripe fruit. You could also include yoghurt, cashew cream or freshly-made cottage cheese, for it goes well with acid and sub-acid fruit.

The ideal is to make the fruit meal your breakfast, and interchange the protein and starch meals at lunch and dinner according to your daily activities. (See the meal planner in Chapter 17. It will help you switch over to compatible meals which follow good FOOD COMBINING principles, until you get used to this new method of eating.)

6
Maintaining the Acid-Alkaline Balance

Without a doubt, your life changes in the most profound way when you eat more alkaline-forming foods. That's because everyone needs a proper ratio of alkaline to acid in their body chemistry to be truly healthy. The pH of 'normal' blood alkalinity in a healthy individual is between 7.35 and 7.45 (i.e. slightly alkaline).

Don't be confused when you see 'pH'. It is simply a scale from 0–14 that measures the acidity/alkalinity of substances. On this scale 0–7 is acid (0 being the most acid) and 7–14 is alkaline (14 being the most alkaline). In other words, all acids have pHs lower than 7, and the lower the number, the more acidic the substance. All alkalis (also called bases) have pHs higher than 7, and the higher the number, the more alkaline.

Pure water has a pH of 7 and is said to be neutral. Saliva in the mouth should be 7 and neutral when not activated by food. An active stomach is 2–5 (acidic) and the small intestine can vary between 5–9 (mild acid to alkaline).

Dr Dudley d'Auverge Wright, in his book *Foods for Health and Healing* says that normal alkalinity of body fluids is the most favourable for the correct action of vitamins. Research groups in America and Sweden have made an even more exciting discovery: when your diet is more than 60 per cent alkaline you receive a tremendous emotional lift. You feel brighter and more energetic. And all obsessive eating and drinking habits improve. Apparently you are more able to give up smoking easily.

Researchers Professor Stanley Schachter in the United States of America and Dr Are Waerland of Sweden were among the first to research the way in which food affects the brain and emotions. This alkaline research is very exciting because it explores how food affects not only health, but the emotions, too. Alkaline foods appear to have the extraordinary ability to 'damp down' obsessive patterns.

I am not suggesting that the psychological reasons behind overweight, or drinking too much, and smoking, just go away. However, I do believe that by making this dietary changeover you can give yourself a chance of fighting back to good health and dealing with life's problems.

So that you can quickly identify what I mean by alkaline foods and acid foods, here is a short shopping list. (A more comprehensive list of common foods, their nutritive value and properties is contained in chapter 20).

- Alkaline-forming foods are all vegetables (including potatoes if cooked in their skins and eaten with skins), all salads, all fresh fruits (except plums and cranberries), almond milk, millet and buckwheat.

  It may sound strange that such acid fruits as oranges, lemons and grapefruit are classified as alkaline. More accurately, they are all alkali-forming because after digestion and absorption into the bloodstream they become alkaline.

- Acid-forming foods are all animal proteins such as meat, fish, shellfish, eggs, dairy products, poultry, nuts (except almonds), all starch foods, such as grains, bread, flour and other foods made from cereal starches and sugars, tea, coffee and alcohol. Refined white sugar and flour are especially acid-forming because they have lost, through the refinement process, valuable alkaline minerals such as calcium, magnesium and potassium.

The taste of these foods does not indicate their acidity, however they have an acidic reaction in the body after digestion has taken place.

Symptoms of an Acid/Toxic System

The obvious symptoms of an acid and toxic system are waking up with a furry tongue and bad breath, insatiable hunger, constant fatigue, bad skin tone and irritability. If the system is highly acid there could be emotional mood shifts, ranging from mild to deep depression.

Overcoming an Acid/Toxic System

Naturopaths and food reformers have been saying for decades that the balance of our daily intake should be at least 60/40 per cent in favour of alkaline foods. Many recommend as high as an 80/20 balance. I believe the ideal diet, therefore, is a four-to-one alkali-acid ratio. To get this, the day's meals must include one protein meal only, one starch meal only and one wholly alkaline meal of fruit and vegetables.

If you recognise yourself as having an 'acid' imbalance and you would like to change quickly, here's the best way to do it. Give FOOD COMBINING a chance so that your digestive system can begin to work more efficiently. Switch over to freshly-squeezed fruit and vegetable juices (see also chapter 14). Eat as much vegetables and fruit as you can, and combine other foods properly.

It may really be worth it too because there is information around to suggest that vegetable eaters are more attractive and sexy to their partners! Researchers are finding out more and more about the power of vegetables and fruit. For instance, Dr Max Lake, the Sydney surgeon and oenologist, has evolved the fascinating theory that people who eat fresh carrots, parsley and green, leafy vegetables exude different, more attractive pheronomes — the sex hormones which affect our scent.

Of course, some people find it very difficult to eat raw vegetables. If you haven't been able to do so until now then you have my sympathy. It means that your worn out, weakened digestive enzymes have probably not been trained to cope with much raw food.

At a holistic Health conference in Britain, Dr Harry Howell declared: 'We have bred a generation of people who don't like and cannot tolerate salads and raw vegetables, all because of poor digestion.' He believes that anyone who cannot eat fresh salad foods every day can never achieve full buoyant health and energy and will be much more susceptible to illness. I'm sure he's right. Fruit and vegetables in their natural state are power-packed with plant enzymes, vitamins, minerals, fibre, plant hormones and many other vital nutrients. More of their extraordinary benefits in chapter 14.

Another doctor at the same Holistic Health Conference estimated that 80 per cent of people eating the average Western diet could not tolerate fresh salad vegetables.

By following the FOOD COMBINING guidelines and not drinking with meals, your more numerous and more vigorous digestive enzymes make eating fresh fruit and vegetables a sheer delight. Even if you have never been able to tolerate raw salad vegetables, you will find that after a time you can greet them with relish. We have proved this again and again. The time it takes varies depending on how weak and toxic the digestion has become. But starting off with daily juices and proper FOOD COMBINING, the majority of people do make very rapid progress within a few days to a few weeks. The raw foods become an enjoyable complement to cooked dishes. And as the live plant enzymes in fresh fruits and vegetables support and encourage the digestive enzymes even more, you begin to assimilate more vitamins, minerals and nutrients from all your food, leading to greater vitality.

The Bitter Principle

Another fascinating theory about food chemistry comes from Dr Peter Theiss, who took a doctorate at the Max Planck Institute in Berlin in neuropharmacology and who later studied herbalism.

He wrote: 'I believe that we are missing an essential ingredient in our nutrition and that element is the bitter principle. All bitter foods are valuable in protecting the liver and they stimulate the natural rhythm of the liver cells.

'Today we have so many sources of pollution which build up in the organs of the body and cause illness. The cause of most illness, I believe, points to toxicity in the body.

'All foods which taste bitter are essential for health. Our ancestors used to instinctively dig in the fields for bitter roots or pluck leaves of other bitter plants when they were sick.'

Surely our livers need protecting more than those of our ancestors. Yet, how many of us now eat artichoke, chicory, watercress, dandelion or raducio on a regular basis?

Nature has given us the ability to distinguish between four distinctly different tastes:

- sweet
- sour
- salty
- bitter.

The papillae—or taste buds are arranged on the tongue in four separate zones. Sweet foods are tasted with the tip of the tongue, bitter at the base. Also our sense of smell is intimately related to our sense of taste.

When we realise that digestion begins with the Ptyalin enzyme released by the stimulated taste buds, we can see that it is essential for our full health that we have a balance between foods to include all four taste types. It is unwise to miss out on any element altogether.

An analysis of the typical Western diet reveals that sweet, sour and salty foods are consumed every day, but that bitter foods are hardly ever eaten, unless you are a heavy black tea drinker (which is not recommended for good health). Indeed bitter tastes have been almost eliminated and sweet tastes substituted. Who now would believe that the 'drink that refreshes' was originally made from the truly refreshing bitter kola nut? Even the almond has had the bitterness removed by selective breeding and cultivation practices.

The taste spectrum has been further reduced in processed foods where sour tastes are also being eliminated. The specially bred gherkins dressing the modern fast food hamburger are light years of taste away from Granny's prize relish. Health suffers in the process, as the concentration of taste sensations leads to salt and sugar addictions.

A bitter taste was an integral part of the diet of indigenous peoples. The Aborigines of northern Australia traditionally ate bitter roots the taste of which is so harsh that it would act on our 'civilised' digestive systems like poison. Yet metabolic disorders were practically unknown among primitive peoples.

The peasant peoples of Europe traditionally took a spring cure of bitter herbs such as dandelion and wild garlic to cleanse their bodies of the toxins accumulated from the restrictive diet during the winter months. Even today it is the custom in many European countries to start a rich meal with a 'digestive' drink compounded from bitter herbs.

So the bitter taste, which was once a vital part of our diet, has now almost vanished in certain countries.

'Yet,' says Dr Theiss, 'the bitter principle in vegetables and herbs activates the liver and helps to get rid of toxins and eliminate poisons from the body. The liver governs the whole process of speeding waste materials from the system.'

But, having said that most people are probably woefully deficient in the bitter principle in nutrition, there are most encouraging signs that things are changing. Curly-headed endive dominates the lettuces; artichokes, chicory, watercress are in most fruit markets just waiting for the shopper.

'Raducio, Eh?', said my local Italian greengrocer, Tony. 'My granny always added a handful of raducio leaves or watercress to the top of every salad. There! That's for the good of your liver, she'd say.' He broke off some fronds of raducio and popped them into his mouth with content.

'Beautiful!'

7
When and How Much to Eat

Up until the last two hundred years or so, it was normal for everyone to sit down to two meals a day. In fact there were many working people who preferred to eat one meal a day.

However, three meals a day, though 'modern', offers a one way ticket to ill health, for it has grown to include between meal snacking called morning and afternoon tea and supper.

In effect we are back to eating one meal which never ends, from breakfast through to bedtime.

The fact that we can and do eat so much is indicative of how affluent we have all become. Finding the mental strength and determination to cut back on our eating habits is not easy when advertising constantly bombards us from television sets and magazines, and when cookbooks compete to outdo each other with superb colour photography showing delectable dishes with mouth-watering ingredients.

Still, for our health's sake we have to begin looking at the quantities we eat and the amount of time we leave between meals. It is a medical fact that the amount we eat can be correlated with how fit we feel. Eat sparingly and well and fitness levels rise. Indulge and gluttonise throughout the day and your body just wants you to sleep or lie around while it deals with the excess food.

Also when we eat too much, we develop what is called 'hidden hunger'. Our modern diet of processed or refined foods promotes hunger pangs, because they lack sufficient nutrients, whereas fresh fruit and vegetables give the body enough nourishment to last comfortably between meals.

We have become, in effect, a nation of food addicts, taking our food with irritating condiments and stimulants, inventing for the novelty, not the goodness, bizarre combinations of ingredients. The result is a growing army of fat people subjected to degenerative disease.

Thanks to advances in medicine we have almost conquered infectious disease; we can replace many worn out organs and select genetically healthy babies. Yet the simple process of overeating is reducing our quality of life. I'm sure that was not the intention when technology made food more abundant to everyone and life less of a battle for survival.

Dr Felix Oswald notes that for more than a thousand years, the one meal habit was the rule in Greece and Rome, both of which kept large armies of men, who could march for days under a load of iron (besides clothes and provisions) stopping only at night for food and sleep. Their stamina in battle was legendary. We now know that it is far easier not to eat while doing physical work, than to begin eating, when the natural inclination is to rest and allow proper digestion.

At the height of the Empire, most Romans, even those from the upper and middle classes, preferred to eat two meals a day. For breakfast they had a glass of water. At midday they ate fruit and cold meat, while the biggest meal was eaten in the evening after work.

Among the wealthy this late meal was a sumptuous affair with wine, pickled sow's udder, oysters, and roasted meats sprinkled with honey and poppy seed and dried fruit.

The working classes and slaves had simple grains and fruits.

The sense in eating less often is obvious. It gives the stomach and intestines time for rest periods. Most people in Western societies eat virtually non stop, which means our digestive systems are in constant use.

At Hopewood we serve three meals a day, but food for each meal is properly combined. We serve a light fruit breakfast at 9 am, a starch or protein lunch at 12.30 pm and a starch or protein dinner at 6 pm. This gives people a balanced food programme each day, namely a fruit meal, a starch-based meal and a protein meal.

The times that these meals are served and the content of each meal are important, because they make it as easy as possible to digest food.

We aim, when planning our meals, to give our guests the chance to rest their stomachs. Fruit in the morning is easily digested so that the stomach is ready, willing and able to tackle lunch.

Lunch is the largest meal of the day, because this is when you need the food most and you are most active.

Dinner is light as this means that during the night the digestive process is well and truly completed and the stomach is able to rest before the morning breakfast begins the cycle all over again. This helps the cleansing process, (you do most of your inner cleansing at night when you are resting). It also enables you to get a better night's sleep. Have you ever wondered by you sometimes have trouble sleeping when you eat heavy foods late at night? It's because your digestive system is keeping you awake because of the excessive demands you have placed on it.

On Hopewood's method of compatible foods, served in small amounts, with at least three hours between meals, and a long overnight period of rest, we have found that guests improve their vitality and energy in remarkably short periods of time.

It is an interesting fact, that when we don't fill ourselves with heavy, badly combined foods, the stomach adjusts, releasing energy for other activities, which would normally be used during digestion.

For perfect health the stomach and intestines should not be required to work simultaneously. They must follow one another. But how can this occur unless we put sufficient time between our meals and be realistic about the quantities we consume at each mealtime.

Why do we put ourselves through so much discomfort which goes against our common sense and natural instinct? Because we are conditioned social animals. We want to be part of the herd, fully accepted by the company we seek.

You must have noticed how a person who doesn't drink, eat meat or party on till late at night, is often ridiculed by members of his or her social circle, with names such as 'spoilsport' or 'wowser'.

Against such criticsm, you have to be a strong self-nurturing and self-loving individual, willing to swim against the tide, buoyed by the knowledge that in the long term what you are doing is in your best interests.

Believe me, this isn't generally a tough road to follow. On a day-to-day basis, you will feel so much better than those who over indulge.

Sadly, there are few of us when young, who have the strength or determination to act in this way, until we create the excuse of illness. We are in effect willing to pay the price of ill health to be accepted.

I hope that times are changing and that more and more young people will realise that the price they pay is too expensive. The sheer cost of our health system is finally forcing those in power to look critically at old age with its chronic ill health. They are asking: 'Can't this be changed?'

Think about it. Your body needs you. It needs you to nurture and care for it throughout life, not just when it finally looks like giving up on you.

How to Eat

As I said, there is a slow change in attitudes. The art of good eating through FOOD COMBINING is beginning to be recognised, which is why you are reading this book. By feeding the body well, in appropriate amounts, and at suitable intervals, we can produce health and vigour and avoid fatness, toxicity, flatulence, heartburn, and long term ill-health.

The first rule is a simple one. *Eat only when hungry!*

If you do not experience hunger even after missing a few meals or after eating lightly for a few days, chances are you need to undergo a cleansing programme (see Chapter 8). If this is the case consult a practitioner experienced in natural health and cleansing.

When the body requires food it will signal this fact and not by excessive gnawing pain, irritability and the shakes. Genuine hunger is a delightful feeling; the saliva glands release juices into the mouth and you feel an expectation and excitement at the thought of food.

It is doubtful if you have spent your life on refined and processed foods, that you have ever experienced genuine hunger. That's because these processed foods are addictive and leave the body starving for genuine nourishment.

Genuine hunger is a pleasant light-hearted state which alerts you to the need for food. If food is unavailable the sensation will disappear until a more appropriate time.

Why not experiment with yourself. Perhaps two meals a day is right for you, with a drink of fruit or vegetable juice at breakfast. If you like a heavy meal in the evening, eat it as early as possible. Forget the sophisticated habit of 'eating late'. It may be pleasant to sit and linger over a late evening meal, but it's your health which is at stake here.

Once you feel pleasantly full, don't eat further. Eat just enough to satisfy your feelings of genuine hunger. Leave food on your plate if necessary. We are lucky to have abundant food, don't over eat because you are guilty about all those poor people in the Asian sub-continent with just a handful of rice to keep them alive. Overeating won't help them, and more importantly it will make you so unproductive you won't have any good ideas on how to improve the world so we can all eat well together.

When you have indigestion, drink herb tea and put up with the discomfort, then make a vow not to abuse your stomach again. Antacids are short term cures and more detrimental to your health in the long term. Use a hot water bottle if your stomach is in pain. The heat will help ease the discomfort.

Lie down and rest. Any activity puts a further strain on the body when it is in pain. Allow the body to deal with the problem as quickly as it can. It can't do that if you are moving around.

Don't eat the next meal after an indigestion attack. Allow the stomach and intestines to fully process the food and then rest before another morsel passes your lips.

8
Detoxification

At Hopewood, while we are introducing people to the principles of FOOD COMBINING, we suggest that they 'cleanse' or 'detoxify' their system first. This really is a vital and necessary process that goes hand in hand with dietary changes because it simply means that we get rid of the build up of toxins stored in our bodies and start again 'clean'.

We cleanse our bodies internally and naturally every day of our lives. However, for many people the sheer volume of toxins they are ingesting and breathing exceeds their ability to get rid of them. This is a particular problem for people affected by high levels of stress and who don't exercise on a regular basis.

It's easy to check whether you have a toxic or acidic system:

- Are you constantly low on energy?
- Do you wake up with a furry tongue or a 'metallic' taste in your mouth?
- Do you have frequent headaches?
- Do you have poor skin tone?
- Do you have dry or lifeless hair?
- Do you have joint and muscular aches and pains?
- Do you remain stubbornly overweight, no matter how you 'starve' yourself?

If your system is particularly toxic and acidic, and you feel constantly tired and likely to be depressed, cleansing may take up to two weeks, coupled with changes in diet, to sweep most of the toxins out of your already overloaded system.

It does seem to have become rather fashionable to worry about detoxifying ourselves, as we are alerted to the ever-increasing pollution that is in the air we breathe, the water we drink, the food we eat and is a result of the increasing volumes of medications we take. Perhaps detoxifying our bodies is the only real way we can make a contribution to the environment. Because there are some who reason that if we clean up ourselves, we'll carry the process through into the world and vice versa.

We are told that the body is a resistant and adaptable mechanism. If this is correct, then detoxifying it on a regular basis is like oiling and greasing a car. It will keep it in good working order longer.

The detox principle is based on the theory that if the body is allowed to rest, cleanse and rejuvenate, then it has a chance to remove the waste, chemical residues and other damaging foreign materials which collect in the cells, organs and bloodstream. If these pollutants are removed frequently there is little build up.

It is argued by many practitioners today that the build up of waste products reduces the body's ability to remain healthy. Toxins can compromise our immune system, respiratory system, lymphatic system, in fact all the systems which maintain our good health. When health is adversely affected in this way, it reduces the potential of the body to prevent acute, chronic and degenerative disease.

Cleansing and fasting are not new ideas. They've been practised for centuries by religious groups and by people who believe that abstinence from food for a day or two leads to clearer thinking and a healthier, more active, physical body.

So what is the difference between cleansing and fasting? Very little, except in modern terminology. Cleansing means the body is doing its house cleaning on light meals and juices. Fasting, traditionally, means abstaining from all food for a period of time, drinking only water.

The rate of cleansing can be varied by altering the intake of food. Fasting on water only usually brings about the strongest rate of cleansing. Juice dieting and/or light meals that are properly combined without much in the way of concentrated proteins or starches, also promote cleansing.

As a general rule of thumb, the more restricted the programme, the more strongly the person will cleanse internally. A word of warning though. You should never contemplate doing a strong cleansing programme without first consulting a practitioner who is experienced in supervising such programmes. It is also best to follow a cleansing programme away from your daily routine, preferably at a place where you can totally rest.

At the Hopewood Health Centre, where cleansing is a vital part of our healing programme, we offer juice and light meal cleansing programmes, as well as water cleansing programmes. But I've found most people who are not familiar with the idea of giving food a miss for several days in order for the body to rest and rejuvenate, seem to find the juice programme or light meals a comforting introduction to the concept of cleansing.

After watching literally thousands and thousands of people undergo cleansing programmes, it appears people these days are less able to tolerate the stronger water cleansing programmes. I discussed this observation with the Hopewood practitoners and in particular with one of the founders of the Centre, Mrs Madge Cockburn, who has more wisdom about natural health than anyone else I've met. It appears that the stronger cleansing programmes are more difficult now because we have greater levels of waste products to dredge out.

At Hopewood, we prepare our guests for cleansing by giving them properly combined fruit and vegetables. Fruit only is usually served as their last solid meal. As I have said in earlier chapters, fruit is easily digested and passes quickly through the body.

By the next morning the body is rested and ready for the stronger cleansing programme to begin. Five juices a day are given at intervals of every three hours from 8 am through to 8 pm. The juices vary according to the practitioners' recommendations. If the person has digestive problems and would rather avoid strong juices such as orange and grapefruit, they have a choice of milder apple or watermelon. Chlorophyll and vegetable juices are also given during the day so that the five juice treatment can be both varied and complimentary.

While the body is receiving only juice, it proceeds to go about its spring-cleaning duties. Energy is not tied up in the digestive process. The juices pass very quickly through the system leaving the body to pull on its reserves of toxins stored in the fatty tissues, often around the legs and waist.

The body is a very efficient machine. It is quickly regenerative if given a chance. You must have noticed how quickly you can heal a cut or boil, if there is no infection and your body is in healthy working order. Conversely look how difficult it is for the body to deal with a wound when it is run down, fatigued and battling infection. Regular tender loving care is what the body yearns for in order to do its work properly.

During the first day on juices, people who are highly toxic often sleep a lot, find they loose all appetite and develop what is called the 'caffeine withdrawal' headache.

For those who do their preparation properly, eating lots of fresh fruit and vegetables and cutting down on their intake of tea and coffee, the withdrawal is significantly reduced.

Any pain is simply the body's reaction to a drug it is used to consuming on a daily basis, namely caffeine. If you have been drinking eight to ten cups of coffee or tea a day, the headache may persist for two days. It is worth putting up with though because once this initial stage is over you begin to feel wonderful and energetic.

A natural relief for any off colour feelings is to lie down with a hot water bottle behind the neck and knees and a cold towel on the temples. The hot/cold treatment opens and constricts the veins accordingly and is especially helpful to headaches.

It stands to reason that if you have been pouring poisons into your body on a regular basis, you will feel ill while you discharge these wastes. The good news is that it is a very temporary feeling of lethargy and vague illness. The juices work quickly and continue to give some substance while flushing out the system. And the best news is that, as a result of the cleansing, you will gain a sense of wellbeing and vitality that may have been missing from your life for years.

Some people say they can't remember ever having felt so well. Usually the first cleansing programme is the toughest. After that, subsequent cleansing treatments get easier, especially when changes are made at home to improve your lifestyle.

Water cleansing works on the same principle and for some (particularly those who are very overweight) it is more satisfying to know that the body has no digestive process to deal with, while it gets on with the cleansing. Small, regular amounts of filtered rainwater are taken throughout the day and into the night. In fact you are encouraged to drink as much water as you want while not overloading the stomach or straining it in any way.

After the initial cleansing process, you are left feeling light and energetic. But this feeling is short lived during each day, which is why those who are on 'detox' programmes must not do anything too strenuous for too long.

Cleansing not only happens through the kidneys and bowels, but also through other parts of the body designed to assist elimination. The skin is the biggest eliminative organ we have and a lot of toxic materials are shed via the skin. Think how clever the body is. It rids itself of toxins regularly, if needed, when, as a result of a lowered immune system, it catches a cold, develops a fever which sweats the toxins through the skin's pores.

While on a cleansing programme, you are encouraged to use the skin to help the body rid itself of waste. Initially, you will feel the cold easily as the blood is utilised internally to speed up the cleansing process. Take a daily warm bath, keep warm and rest, it soon passes.

Dry skin brushing is another method of speeding the toxins from the skin mantle. This cleansing method requires a vegetable bristle brush which is moved in gentle regular strokes across the body. The skin will turn red as the blood is stimulated to the surface of the skin, but this soon disappears. Dry skin brushing is also a wonderful way to get circulation into those white cellulite areas on the tops of the legs. It brings the blood into the dimpled areas and helps break down the fatty deposits.

Some bloating and flatulence may occur during the first days of cleansing, but this also passes. Loose bowel action is another possible activity the body may employ. This is not something to be anxious about. The fruit juices or water are simply washing faecal matter from the intestinal walls and flushing it out of the system. Bowel inactivity is more the norm.

For some, the nose may start to run. Again this is a way the body has of ridding itself of toxic materials. When the mucous membrane starts discharging, it is simply your body discharging excess toxins which have built up there.

How Long Does Cleansing Take

You probably wonder how long a cleansing programme should take. That depends on your state of health, age and vitality. It does not follow that if you are older you have been storing wastes for longer than a young person and therefore you need weeks to dislodge the toxins.

How long you choose to cleanse depends on your lifestyle and how you feel. You may have modified your way of eating and be feeling simply tired and run down. In which case you probably only need three or four days on a juice diet to rest and revitalise.

If you do only need a short cleanse, chances are you won't have many side effects and your energy will return fairly quickly during the cleansing period.

You may lead an indulgent life, eating fats, starches and proteins in one big mix during every meal. If you are inactive, overweight, constantly tired and lacking energy, if you have a disease which will respond to a nutrition-based programme, then you may need from one to two weeks on juices, or even a water programme for several days, returning to eating via juices and then light salads and fruits.

Whatever your programme, you must remember that if you do follow a cleansing juice or water programme, the number of days you don't eat must correspond with the days you spend returning to normal eating patterns. You can harm your digestive system by jumping from a cleansing fast straight onto heavy meals. Your digestive system has been resting and spring cleaning. It needs to be reintroduced to food slowly via light meals of fresh fruit and steamed vegetables and salads. It is wise to wait even an extra few days, before you introduce the heavier meat proteins and fats.

From this point, to maintain that new found vitality and good feeling, you must be prepared to begin eating fruit each morning on an empty stomach, then during the rest of the day follow FOOD COMBINING guidelines choosing starches, fats and carbohydrates in one meal and your proteins and vegetables in another meal.

Keep in mind that any time you alter your eating habits, your body needs an adjustment period. This adjustment may leave you feeling initially out of sorts. It is only a temporary discomfort. The body must learn to accept good eating habits just the same way it learnt to accommodate your bad eating habits. And the elimination of a good deal of toxicity from your body may take months or years. But I promise you that within days you will begin losing weight and you will feel enormously energetic and vibrant.

I have often been told at Hopewood that a two week rest and cleansing programme does more than any month long holiday. That is because on holiday you are simply unwinding—letting go of the stress and sleeping well. At Hopewood you are cleansing as well and the combination of all three is an extremely powerful rejuvenator.

9
Losing Weight — Feeling Great

This is one of the most marvellous benefits of the FOOD COMBINING way of life. Your body just smoothly and gradually adjusts to its ideal weight. For some people the flab and bulges roll off like excess baggage.

Again, there are many good reasons why FOOD COMBINING succeeds so brilliantly where so many diets end in misery and failure.

For a start, you're eating the same amount of food, but containing fewer kilojoules. Just to give a few examples: a plateful of pasta topped with spinach sauce has only half the kilojoules of pasta and bolognaise sauce with meat. Muesli served with pear or apple juice is much less fattening than eating it with milk or soymilk. Soya beans cooked in tomato sauce and served with tofu and zucchini have far fewer kilojoules than baked beans on toast and are just as satisfying. Chicken served with a medley of extra vegetables, lightly steamed, will satisfy the most voracious appetite and still be less calorific than the traditional meat with potato or rice and two vegetables.

You can heap your plate with broccoli, green beans, corn on the cob, asparagus, cabbage, Brussels sprouts — they won't add weight. In fact, some vegetables, such as Brussels sprouts, cabbage, zucchini, celery, tomato and asparagus (I give a complete list in Chapter 20) are so low in kilojoules that you can literally eat as much as you like of them.

As an accurate comparison consider this: one and a half cups of cauliflower contain 180 kilojoules; one cup of carrots 190 kilojoules; one cup of green cabbage has only 113 kilojoules; one cup of Brussels sprouts a mere 210 kilojoules. On the other hand one small chicken quarter, baked or grilled with skin contains 350 kilojoules. One lamb chop with all fat removed is 850 kilojoules, with fat left on it's a whopping cholesterol-laden 2000 kilojoules. And an average big sausage is around 700 kilojoules, while one average slice of ham varies from 170 to 330 kilojoules.

There is an absolutely fundamental reason why you slim down with such ease and enjoyment following the FOOD COMBINING system of eating. With an improved digestion, your body is now assimilating—perhaps for the first time in years—all the vitamins, minerals and nutrients and amino acids it needs to renew cells and for proper metabolism. As amino acid expert, natural therapist Sean Goss points out, 'You may have been eating lots of food, but very little will have been reaching the target.'

Our bodies seem to have an inherent wisdom. Robbed of essential nutrients and amino acids by poor gastric secretions, the appestat—the appetite control centre in the brain—goes on 'red alert'. A message flashes down the biochemical pathways. 'Eat More Food Quickly'. Hunger pangs are felt, sometimes quite soon after a full meal, and so we feel compelled to go on eating more and more without feeling satisfied.

For most of us, weak enzyme action means a constant hunger and the urge to overeat. When they're working properly the digestive enzymes are mighty catalysts which make every mouthful of food more satisfying to the hunger pangs.

After a diet, your body is even more starved of essential elements. This is why, of course, so many of us break out into a full-tilt binge and eat something like an entire crusty French loaf or a whole box of chocolates. Then we go through the miserable cycle of self-hatred, diet and binge yet again. In any case, diets don't seem to work. They are usually deprivation programmes people follow for a limited period of time. When they have reached their goal weight (or when they can't stand it any longer), they go back to the same food and lifestyle that caused the problems in the first place. What I am suggesting in this book is a permanent and enjoyable change in the way we live, that will maintain a slim, healthy body.

As we've seen, when protein is eaten at the same time as starch food, it can sit in the stomach for about eight hours and take twenty hours to pass through the intestines. On the standard three meals a day plan, the food is still waiting to be digested when another meal comes along. The food is quite likely to putrefy or ferment (which is not a pleasant thought), so that there is a toxic load on board and one that is keeping you overweight.

Because digestion time is greatly increased without FOOD COMBINING, the food sits in your stomach all day long not being properly digested. Dr Herbert M. Shelton, who researched FOOD COMBINING for over 40 years estimated a heavy, badly combined meal could take ten hours just to leave the stomach.

Anyone who suffers indigestion, heartburn, or gas and wind should know that food is fermenting or putrefying in the digestive tract. And since antacids sell by the millions in all Western countries, that means a high percentage of us are experiencing these symptoms.

Since improperly digested food is hard to eliminate too, many have to resort to laxatives as well.

With several meals under your belt awaiting digestion, bariatrician (an expert on slimming) Ronald A. Butterworth says that colonic content alone can account for between one and 3½ kilograms in weight. This is why the first advice he gives people who go to him to learn to eat successfully, is to throw away the weighing scales. He explains how, given this situation, it is useless to climb on the scales each morning and sigh over one or two kilos lost or regained.

That's an astonishing thought when you think about it. We can actually carry around more than 3 kilograms of poorly digested food awaiting elimination. No wonder it's hard to achieve a flat stomach when it is literally weighed down by that burden.

The toxic load is the reason, too, for the persistent extra weight of the small percentage of people who protest, quite honestly, that they eat very little. What they do eat stays around a long time and builds fat because of an extremely slow metabolism.

Further, it appears our bodies protect us from fat soluble toxins by storing them in cells surrounded by fat. Hence the cellulite problem which is experienced by many women living on a Western diet.

With FOOD COMBINING, for the first time, perhaps, losing weight becomes a pleasure.

10
The Need to be Active

FOOD COMBINING and eating quality foods are much more effective if you combine this with some form of physical activity.

Health and vigour are synonymous because vigorous people are healthy people. That's because activity (notice I avoid the dreaded word exercise) is vital to the health of your bones, muscles and, more important, your heart muscle.

Your whole body functions so much better when you are fit. You also have improved feelings of self esteem and a better physical shape. Good food and enjoyable exercise support each other. For example you are less likely to eat junk food when you are aware of your physical health and wellbeing. Conversely, when you are racked with feelings of low self-esteem, you are more likely to adopt 'destructive' habits.

Chances are you have been told too many times that you must exercise. It's a case of the naughty child. If it is said too often, then the child rebels and deliberately does the opposite.

What I'm suggesting here is some form of regular activity such as brisk walking, rebounding on a mini trampoline in your home, bicycling, swimming, running— anything that will give your skin a glow of sweat and elevate your pulse. Ideally you will be looking for a form of exercise that suits you. One that raises your pulse rate for at least 20 minutes to a good training level without overdoing it and one which you can follow at least three times per week.

Check with your practitioner if you have had heart or circulatory problems or if you are in doubt about your ability to undertake an exercise programme. Then select an exercise that appeals to you.

It is good to balance aerobic forms of exercise with activities such as Yoga, Tai Chi or Relaxacise. These pursuits blend together very well our physical and mental components. Whatever form of exercise you feel attracted to, do it and do it regularly.

The more you move your muscles the more you are sending those vital nutrients you have eaten throughout your body and removing waste products. With increased nutrition, there is increased strength.

It is estimated that there are some 600 odd muscles in the body, each of them in need of regular exercise. If you don't believe me go and do something you haven't done for years, such as water skiing, or play a game of tennis. The next day you will be stiff and sore and you will become aware that you have used muscles you probably never thought existed before.

Our muscular system constitutes by weight the bulk of our body (40–50 per cent). If you neglect them, muscles waste and weaken and all function which depends upon the actions of the muscles deteriorates. If you have been in bed constantly for a month, there is wasting and weakness of your muscles. Such a simple experience must convince you how important activity of one kind or another is to your health and, more important, to your feelings of wellbeing!

If you cringe from the word exercise, as many do, think of exercise as a body function. Muscular action is actually a means of pushing the blood and lymph through the tissues of the body. The active muscle needs more blood, which is why action automatically provides an increase in circulation. The contraction of the muscle expresses blood from it. While relaxed, blood is allowed to flow back into it.

Heavy breathing in the chest also helps increase the muscular contractions, thus increasing the rate of blood and lymph flow.

Blood is propelled by the heart, but so interrelated are heart and blood that it is the accumulation of blood in the chambers of the heart that trigger its pulsations. If we are never sufficiently active to create a rapid flow of blood through the heart, its actions become feeble and its strength and size decrease. Every part of the body is linked in its actions to all the rest. Nowhere is this more apparent than in the circulatory system when the body is active.

Our bodies were designed for a life of constant activity. And they function best when we give them regular exercise. Normal everyday movements are not sufficient exercise for your muscles. Even a labourer needs to exercise, because not all his muscles are being used on the job. Job related activities do not always raise the pulse rate to a high enough level, nor for a long enough continuous duration to gain real benefits. That is why you can find a lot of labourers who are strong, but not fit, or really healthy. As our jobs become more specialised, so we use less of our muscular system.

Muscles have only two actions and these are contraction and relaxation. It's as simple as that. Exercise or activity is just the alternate contraction and relaxation of the muscles. You don't have to run a marathon or end up exhausted after a one hour aerobic workout. The body doesn't appreciate being overtaxed. You have to build on your exercise plan day-by-day so that increasing exercise becomes a pleasure—something you and your body look forward to and need, even crave as you get healthier.

In fact as your health improves through FOOD COM-

BINING I would not be surprised if you suddenly get more active without really planning to. That's what happens when the body feels good. It encourages movement. When it is sick it encourages no action so that it is not distracted from its healing work.

Don't feel guilty if you don't have much activity in your life at present. Work on your diet, and let the action flow from that. What I am saying is be aware that you can't have health without activity.

Try to do some form of exercise in the early morning. That is when your body feels rested, when your stomach is empty and when the air is freshest. Take several deep breaths and set aside time for you to get those muscles moving.

The point to remember as you build a healthier, happier body, is that you are looking to revitalise your body and exercise is as important as good food.

11
Water — Beware!

We have all been educated to know that drinking enough water is essential for real health and vitality. And if you are going to build your energy supplies through good FOOD COMBINING, you must also pay attention to your fluid intake.

The question is how much water is enough?

The logical answer is drink as much as is required to satisfy your thirst. Nature gave us the perfect guide, but most of us have to some degree distorted it by eating salty foods, very sweet foods, spices, condiments, greasy fatty dishes and other highly concentrated foods which are not true thirst indicators, but rather irritations to the mouth and stomach. What about tea, coffee and wine? Sad to say they are natural dehydrants which deplete the body's reserves of water.

Water will not stop this kind of thirst. It will simply weaken the digestive juices and interfere with the digestion, doing more harm than good. If you insist on eating and drinking these kinds of products which make you feel 'thirsty' then sip half a glass of water slowly. If you still feel you want more water, ignore your desire, it will pass.

By contrast, people who eat more fresh fruits and vegetables get more water from their food than those who eat a lot of processed foods that contain no natural juices, and they, therefore feel less thirsty.

Until recently, there was an accepted 'rule of thumb'

that the best amount of water was six to eight glasses a day. Now that is being challenged by experts.

'After all', says Dr Abram Hoffer, 'the amount of water a 95 kilo man needs will differ from that of a 55 kilo woman. It's a question of finding your own best level.'

Dr Hoffer is an extraordinary researcher: a medical doctor, psychiatrist, nutritionist and orthomolecular scientist, he was one of those responsible for introducing the 'water wagons' into Canadian hospitals. He has the riveting habit of opening his lectures with this statement: 'Before I start, I can tell that you won't remember much of what I say because most of you haven't drunk enough water!' There is a slight pause while delegates rush to the water containers. Then Dr Hoffer goes on to explain that without sufficient daily water the brain cells actually begin to shrivel and the short and long term memory are both affected.

In Canadian hospitals, doctors noticed a marked improvement in many mental patients and especially in eldery people who had been classified as suffering from senile dementia, when they began to drink more water. Apparently the brain cells have a tremendous capacity for revival under the influence of water.

I think it's fair to say that most of us do not drink nearly enough water. However, avoid drinking with meals. This is important. While food is being eaten, large quantities of digestive juices are poured into the stomach. If water or other fluids are taken at the same time, the digestive juices are diluted and cannot work properly. Water passes out of the stomach relatively quickly and carries the digestive juices out with it. Deprived of these juices, digestion is slowed and fermentation and putrefaction follows.

Drinking and eating together also lead to 'bloating' of the stomach. If you treat the stomach in this way over many years you can develop chronic indigestion, gastritis, ulcers, and even worse problems.

Also when you drink with food you suppress those natural feelings of satisfaction—that you have eaten enough. Consequently you tend to overeat. A classic example of this is drinking beer with salted peanuts. One stimulates the other so that you can go on consuming beer and peanuts long after your appetite is satisfied.

It is alright to drink water fifteen minutes before a meal, however, other fluids contain dissolved substances which take longer to pass through the system, so they should be drunk at least half an hour before a meal, and preferably one hour.

Avoid drinking after a meal as long as food is still digesting in the stomach. A typical meal takes three to four hours, so wait at least two hours for that cup of herbal tea or cereal coffee.

What about soup you ask? Unless it is extremely thick, soup is actually a fluid and is better eaten at least one hour before the main course.

Finally remember that very hot and very cold fluids interfere with digestion. The optimum temperature for digestion is close to body temperature. Take cold and hot drinks when the stomach is empty or very close to it.

Tapwater Can Make You Sick!

Now that we have established that we probably all need to drink more water and preferably between meals, the question is: what kind of water? The answer is emphatically—not straight tapwater.

Research-based facts are emerging all the time to indicate that tapwater may be the cause of many sicknesses, and of premature ageing. Tapwater contains a lot of 'nasties', some of them very nasty indeed. It can contain organic chlorine compounds such as pesticides and disinfectant by-products, and metals in amounts well in excess of accepted safety limits.

Of course our domestic water has to be disinfected to protect us from water-borne pathogens. The trouble is, that the major water purifier, chlorine, has emerged as one of the major health hazards of our age. Chlorine is what gives the acrid and pungent taste to our water. It is a powerful germ killer. Unfortunately, chlorine also presents some side effects which can be nothing short of devastating to our health.

The water authorities adjust the chlorine supply according to the season and to counteract the particular nasties which have leached into the system, such as bird contamination of open reservoirs and seepage over leaking pipes. So there are 'chlorine high' periods. Unfortunately, for certain sensitive people, taking a bath or shower during a 'chlorine high' period, may knock their immune system down for days or weeks.

The list of illnesses that chlorine alone can contribute to should send us rushing for the nearest water filter or bottled mineral water.

A Sydney doctor, Mark Donohoe has found that toxic chlorine by-products in tapwater are a major cause of Chronic Fatigue Syndrome (CFS). This is a baffling and utterly debilitating condition which is affecting thousands of men and women. The major symptoms are persistent fatigue—no matter how much rest; joint pains, memory loss and chronic depression. And Dr Donohoe says it is quite possible to have Chronic Fatigue Syndrome and not be aware you have it.

Chlorine's health-destroying properties do not stop there. In New Jersey, USA, Dr Ronald Pataki conducted a study and found that the severity of heart disease among people over fifty years of age correlated directly with the quantities of chlorinated tapwater they were accustomed to drinking. Dr Pataki found that chlorinated water destroyed Vitamin E and Vitamin C. Since Vitamin E is essential for healthy hearts and good circulation, this is a daily strike against good health. Vitamin C, of course, is essential for every good cellular function, and resistance to disease.

Vitamin C and garlic are natural chelating agents which bond onto chlorine and heavy metals like lead and copper and excrete them out of the body. Make sure there are generous quantities of these nutrients in your FOOD COMBINING diet of fresh fruit, vegetables, nuts and seeds.

Staying Younger and Better Looking

Without a doubt, if you take the trouble to set aside some filtered or otherwise unchlorinated water to wash your face, your skin will positively blossom. Chlorine has been shown to react with the natural lipid layer of the skin to form toxic chlorinated compounds. Several eminent doctors believe that regular exposure to chlorinated water accelerates the ageing process.

Of course, I am not suggesting that all signs of ageing will be wiped out when you stop using tapwater. You also need to eat properly combined and compatible amounts of fresh cooked and uncooked food, get adequate amounts of quality exercise and rest and find your way to better manage the stress of modern living.

However, French tests have shown that small surface wrinkles 'plump out' and appear to disappear with pure water therapy and a healthy simple diet. Your eyes regain the sparkle they may not have had for many years. For younger people, pure water applied to the skin and drunk daily has been shown to help with problematic skin conditions such as acne and eczema.

It is quite fascinating that two such varied cultures as the French and the Japanese have come to the same conclusion: that chlorinated water must be avoided at all costs to preserve young looking skin. And that 'pure water' must be drunk daily and sprayed on the skin to stay young and good looking.

In Japan, the water is often de-chlorinated by a number of different filtration products such as we now have in Australia, plus an intriguing old tradition of putting special volcanic stones for eight hours in a water jar. Hardworking Japanese women in their forties who wash their faces with this 'stone water' are said to have supple, superbly toned, unlined skin.

A French dermatologist working with the Evian Company conducted tests over several years and concluded that most dry and premature ageing skin is due to dehydration—lack of water—as well as lack of protection from the ultra violet rays of the sun. Another French dermatological team made the interesting discovery that when we don't drink enough water, particularly women on unbalanced diets, the skin suffers most. In one test they held, on a water restricted diet, the skin lost nine per cent of its water after eight days, whereas the muscles only lost about two per cent.

Is it any wonder that constant dieters look haggard?

Tapwater Can Make You Fat!

No, it is not fanciful to say that drinking chlorinated water can make you put on weight. As chlorine kills all bacteria it comes in contact with, it attacks the friendly essential microflora in the system too.

Chlorine is a powerful oxidising agent which readily destroys enzymes, certain vitamins and beneficial bacteria.

When these are overpowered our internal balance is destroyed.

American researcher Natasha Trenev sums it up succinctly: Tapwater contains chlorine and pesticide residues and other undesirable chemicals so frequently in the news. Since chlorine is used to kill bad bacteria, these chemicals will certainly kill the friendly bacteria in our digestive tract as well.

And when that happens, you feel hungrier. There is no doubt that when your digestive enzymes and friendly bacteria are under attack, ordinary amounts of food no longer satisfy the hunger pangs.

At the start of this book I discussed the possibility that you may not be able to tolerate raw food with all its remarkable benefits if you have been on a diet of refined and processed foods for years. And that you may now find you go on eating long after most people have stopped. Apart from feeling constantly hungry, you may well have bloating and indigestion, which seems very unfair.

The reason is, of course, that the disturbed digestive enzymes and friendly and not-so-friendly bacteria are playing up. If the friendly bacteria have been overcome, there is a perfect chance you have *candida albicans*, a yeast overgrowth, which takes hold of your body and makes life miserable.

So what is the answer? Buy the best water filter you can afford which takes out all the chlorine, fluoride and pesticides. Or drink pure water which can be purchased through health food stores.

But most of all, learn to enjoy drinking pure water!

To Obtain Pure Water
I believe it pays everybody to obtain water for drinking

which has had all contaminants removed from it, especially fluorine, chlorine and aluminium. This can be done by collecting rainwater which is then filtered as we do at Hopewood; by buying bottled purified water; or by having a purifier attached to your kitchen tap.

Boiled water is quite inadequate because the five minutes of boiling kills harmful bacteria and viruses, plus it removes most of the chlorine, but it has no effect on fluoride, aluminium, heavy metals or other substances in ionic form, other than to concentrate them and make the problem worse.

If you live in the city, rainwater is usually so polluted it is better to drink tap water. But in the country, at least 50 kilometres from big city (more on a highway), it is the best and most economical water to drink. Be aware though, that aerial sprays used in agriculture can contaminate rainwater tanks in country areas.

Bottled purified water is an excellent source of high purity water, but the cost may be a factor which makes it impossible for you to consider. Purifying your own drinking water is probably the most economical long term solution and there are several types of water filters to consider:

Activated carbon filters remove odours, chlorine, pesticide residues and many organic chemicals such as chloroform. Their effectiveness for fluorides and toxic metals is generally not good, although it varies with the brand. For true efficiency the activated carbon must be replaced frequently to avoid bacterial contamination.

Silver carbon matrix filters are activated carbon impregnated with silver to inhibit the growth of bacteria. *Ion-exchange* or *ionised resin filters* mean that the water passes through a column of special resin impregnated with positively and negatively charged ions. Theoretically, this removes everything that activated carbon doesn't, that is toxic metals, nitrates and fluoride.

Reverse osmosis purifiers contain a large area of porous membrane which allows only small molecules, mainly water, to pass through and the trapped impurities are flushed away. Reverse osmosis units are generally expensive, but they are the most effective in removing a wide range of impurities.

Ceramic filters contain ceramic material with very fine holes and may also have silver or carbon. They do not remove all of the impurities and no fluoride at all.

Distillers remove most impurities, including fluoride and chlorine, but not all of the organic compounds such as pesticide and detergent residues. Distillers are expensive, bulky and slow and consume energy so that they end up relatively expensive to run.

12
Bountiful Bioflora

The food we eat consists of many complex compounds. However these compounds cannot pass into the body's metabolic processes in their original forms, but must first be broken down into simple molecules by enzymatic action. They are then absorbed into the body through the intestinal walls before they can be metabolised in the cells to create new body tissue or energy.

The absorption of the nutrient molecules begins in the small intestine with the aid of thousands of millions of bacteria, the biological bacterial flora or bioflora for short.

As well as preparing the nutrients for absorption, the bioflora fulfill another role as the body's first line of defence against dangerous organisms consumed with food. A film of bioflora covers the intestinal mucous mebranes, forming a barrier which in ideal conditions cannot be overcome by infectious pathogens.

If the bioflora is destroyed or the balance is altered, the intestines can malfunction, which may be associated with illness such as lowered resistance to infection, constipation, diverticulitis, bronchial asthma, allergy, heart disease and cancer.

The damage may be caused by poisons such as nicotine, alcohol and caffeine, by antibiotics, whether medically prescribed or as residues in our food resulting from modern farming, by other medical drugs and by incorrect nutrition and eating habits.

The enzymatic problems with milk have already been

discussed. The bioflora also have problems with improperly combined milk. What should happen is that the small intestine secretes the enzyme lactase which digests the milk sugar, lactose (a disaccharide) and turns it into glucose and galactose (a monosaccharide) which is easily absorbed. Late and insufficient secretion of lactase means that much of the undigested lactose passes into the large intestine where it is fermented by the resident bacteria (which is different from that in the small intestine).

The lactic acid and gas resulting from the ferment causes flatulence and even diarrhoea in the body. The balance of the bioflora in the intestines is also upset and the assimulation of nutrients is diminished.

The rules of FOOD COMBINING require milk to be consumed, if at all, on its own so that there is no delay in the secretion of lactase. However, it is quite common among adults of some races, eg Japanese, Phillipino, Negroes, to have little or no lactase, which greatly reduces their ability to digest and assimilate dairy products.

The averge human body contains about 1.6 kilograms of bioflora, both 'friendly' and 'pathogenic'. The most important of the friendly bacteria are *Lactobacillus acidophilus* and *Bifidobacteria*.

The *Bifidobacteria* are the most prevalent bioflora in healthy individuals and reside primarily in the large intestine. They acidify the bowel, preventing *candida albicans* from changing to the pathogenic fungal form and assist intestinal peristalsis, thus relieving constipation. They also aid the liver in detoxifying the bloodstream and improving protein synthesis.

Lactobacillus acidophilus bacteria populate the small intestine and so form the vanguard ahead of *Bifidobacteria*. They produce acidophilin, a natural antibiotic which destroys some common pathogens.

They also assist in maintaining the *Bifidobacteria* and assist in suppressing *candidiasis*.

Lactobacillus acidophilus appears to be the most important friendly intestinal symbiont for those on the standard meat-eating western diet. It does not like to live away from the human gut, so that the problem with taking supplements is to ensure that the acidophilus in them is still viable. Some yoghurts and cultured milks now contain acidophilus, but are better consumed as fresh as possible. Direct supplements must be kept refrigerated.

In addition to the indigenous flora, other transient friendly bioflora can exist within the gastrointestinal system. The specific bacteria will depend on the diet and other lifestyle factors. One such bacteria is *lactobacillus bulgaricus*, present in most natural yoghurts. Others are present in sauerkraut and fermented beet juice and generally in all enzyme rich natural foods.

Enzymes
Enzymes are sensitive to a wide variety of chemical substances and are easily destroyed by them. Great numbers of drugs therefore are enzyme destructive. For example salivary Amylase is inactivated by acids and Pepsin is inactivated by soda and other strong alkalines.

When drugs are taken, it is impossible to know in advance how much they will interfere with the action of enzymes. We do know that organic enzymes are easily destroyed by heat and inactivated by inappropriate pH levels.

Secretion, or the production of enzymes by the various glands in the body, is an essential part of the function of nutrition. We can divide enzyme (hormone) secretions into two general classes:

1 those involved in the preparation of food for entrance into the bloodstream, and
2 those involved in utilising prepared materials after they enter the bloodstream.

The first of these are digestive secretions, the second are endocrine secretions. All secretions are manufactured by digestive and endocrine glands using materials supplied by the blood. This means they are all made from food.

The saliva of the mouth, the gastric juice in the stomach, the pancreatic juice, the intestinal juice and the bile of the liver are all instrumental in digesting food. These juices, except bile (which is really an excretory product) contain one or more enzymes.

Once the digested food enters the bloodstream, digestion ends. But there is still a need for other secretions. They incorporate food into the flesh, blood and bone of the individual. It is at this stage of the process that the hormones secreted by the endocrine glands, are bought to play upon the nutritive processes.

As you can see the body is indeed a finely tuned engine which needs first quality 'oil' to keep it running in superb condition.

You would not abuse a beautiful car or other piece of fine man-made equipment. Why do so with the most magnificent piece of equipment of all—your own body!

13
Yoghurt — Milk of Eternal Life

Amidst daily accounts of doom and gloom about our daily diet, how welcome it is to learn the good news that certain foods can literally do us a power of good.

Yoghurt has now been proven to have exceptional qualities. This fermented milk culture has a particularly interesting history. According to an ancient tradition, an angel revealed to the prophet Abraham the method of making yoghurt.

Cultured milk is produced by the action of bacterial micro-organisms which change the lactose (milk sugar) into lactic acid. The result is an acid curd. The flavour and texture of yoghurt is imparted by a culture made up of *Lactobacillus* organisms.

To many Middle Eastern and Balkan peoples, yoghurt holds the most honoured place on the table. When the French King Francois the First was ailing, he ordered his doctors to find out the secret Balkan formula with the reputation of prolonging youth and vigour. A doctor from Constantinople was sent for immediately and he arrived with his precious yoghurt culture in his pocket. The yoghurt so transformed the King that he named it 'milk of eternal life'.

But it was the Nobel prizewinner, Professor Ilya Metchnikoff, who noted as early as 1908 that Bulgarians and other Balkan people who ate yoghurt daily, lived long and vigorous lives. He was particularly fascinated by the Bulgarian peasants, who, apart from their daily yoghurt, eked out a poor existence, yet lived to ripe old ages. 'They are strong as roots,' he wrote.

Professor Metchnikoff published his findings in his work *The Prolongation of Life* which started the medical interest in yoghurt which has never stopped. Metchnikoff's research convinced him that yoghurt can help our health in four main ways. 'There is no doubt,' he wrote 'that yoghurt has natural antibiotic quality; it is a powerful natural antigermicide which can kill harmful germs; it can help the essential friendly bacteria; and it helps the body to manufacture the B vitamins.'

On all counts, modern research has proved Professor Metchnikoff right.

Certainly in FOOD COMBINING terms, yoghurt is gentle on the digestion and can be mixed with protein rich foods, acid/sub-acid fruits and makes a great base for salad dressings. The culture in the yoghurt breaks down the milk so that it is easily digestible, (it is, in fact, already partly digested) unlike milk itself.

A Fine Natural Antibiotic

Eighty years after Professor Metchnikoff's findings, researchers in America used the latest technology to test yoghurt's benefits. In 1988, at the University of Nebraska, Dr Khem M. Shahani and his colleagues found that natural yoghurt cultured with *Lactobacillus acidophilus* and *Lactobacillus bulgaricus* did indeed have both natural antibiotic and strong antibacterial properties. He found that the culture *L. acidophilus* in yoghurt was even strong enough to inhibit the often deadly staphylococcus and streptococcus germs. The yoghurt was shown to retard other toxins, too, and speed them from the system.

Doctors F. Ferrer and L. J. Boyd fed prune whip yoghurt (natural yoghurt with chopped up cooked prunes in juice) to elderly patients with chronic constipation. Not only did that condition improve, but the doctors noted that the general health and skin tone of their patients improved dramatically too.

Helping the 'Good Guys'—the Friendly Microflora

One of the most important and now well proven abilities of this remarkable food is the way in which it helps the 'friendly' bacteria or microflora re-establish themselves.

These friendly bacteria are absolutely essential for full health as I have said in chapter 12. They can be easily disturbed or killed off by such factors as: tapwater, alcohol, stress, antibiotics, all cortisone type drugs, the birth control pill, etc.

Even if you avoid drugs and have not consciously taken antibiotics for years, here's an unpleasant but true thought. As one endocrinologist wrote: 'All meat eaters get a regular dose of the antibiotics which have been fed to the animals. Many of them are fed hormones too, and in some case even steroids are permitted.' The doctor goes on to say that she has seen cases of young boys in puberty developing female characteristics because of the hormones in meat, particularly, in her opinion, chicken whose growth is accelerated so that the birds can be killed and packaged quickly.

Dr Shahani and others have made the fortunate discovery that regular amounts of natural yoghurt help maintain a stable and protective environment for the good intestinal flora and enable them to flourish. Dr Seneca at Columbia University conducted tests which showed that when yoghurt was eaten regularly over a period of months, no other bacteria except friendly ones appeared in test samples. This vindicated Professor Metchnikoff's own tests in the laboratory at the Pasteur Institute in Paris which found exactly the same results. It further convinced the Nobel Prizewinner that much of the body's health is dependent on the health of the intestines.

The good news is that increasing numbers of people who are unable to drink milk through lactose intolerance, or who wish to follow FOOD COMBINING principles, can eat small amounts of fresh yoghurt.

It is best to eat no more than 1 cup of yoghurt every second day as too much yoghurt will introduce too much lactobacillus into the digestive tract and this could be detrimental to our own 'friendly' bacteria.

Natural yoghurt is available today in good health food shops and should be eaten regularly with relish. However, check the quality and brand. Many commercial yoghurts are not made with the 'good' strains and cultures.

It's very easy to make your own yoghurt too, once you have a good culture to start with. This can be obtained from any good natural yoghurt brand.

Just warm the milk, introduce a tablespoon of yoghurt and the culture will turn the milk into yoghurt overnight.

So yoghurt is a magnificent 'health food' with quite remarkable benefits. It certainly helps synthesise the B vitamins and essential enzymes needed for good digestion.

And good digestion is what we are seeking to establish in this book by FOOD COMBINING and restoring common sense to our daily diet.

14
Green Power — the Power of Juice

Plants have a powerful revitalising effect on the body. They are easy to digest and in juice form they pass through the system quickly giving the digestive tract a chance to restore any imbalance.

Welcome news from German scientists researching vegetables and their benefits as natural plant medicine, comes from Nobel Prize winner, Professor Otto Warburn, who announced that certain vegetables were especially rich in the 'redox' effect. This means that these foods have the ability to give life-giving oxygen to every cell in the human body. 'It is the beginning of revitalisation,' says Professor Warburn.

The foods which the German scientists found had such remarkable 'redox' qualities were beetroot, carrot, horseradish. They are some of the top 'green power foods' we use at Hopewood.

Beetroot
The benefits of beetroot as a liver cleanser and tonic is highly appreciated in alternative medicine. Ancient folklore too rates this vegetable very highly indeed.

All over France, men and women who frankly enjoy their wine, set aside one week a year to 'rest the liver'. During this time a wine glass full of raw beetroot juice is drunk each morning on an empty stomach. And then, throughout the day, four more glasses of beetroot juice are taken at intervals.

Beetroot juice or root taken in large amounts medicinally for short periods can sometimes stain the stool or urine, but do not be alarmed by this.

The tonic value of this vegetable was investigated at Warsaw University in the early 1970s, where a control group drank raw beetroot juice daily throughout the three winter months. Researchers found that the group had fewer colds than the national average and that several overweight members also lost weight.

This weight loss is particularly interesting, since beet is rich in natural sugar and usually shunned by slimmers. The answer lies in beetroot's stimulating effect on the liver which metabolises fat cells.

Beetroot has yet more to offer. The green leaves, so often chopped off at the greengrocer's shop are rich in natural hormones related to oestrogen. It becomes clear now why Russian and all Eastern European women have always eaten beetroot leaves, to regulate their hormones and keep them fertile. The leaves are also rich in iron and provide excellent amounts of vitamin A. In fact, beet leaves are one of the richest natural sources of both iron and vitamin A and contain more than three times the amount found in apricots.

In Russia, beetroot soups, salads and juices are used daily to keep the body's resistance high. Russian Borsch is a soup appreciated by gourmets around the world.

Raw beetroot has a distinctive earthy taste, but don't be put off. The Russians have created a delicious way for anyone to learn to love raw beetroot. It is grated very finely and mixed half and half with cooked beetroot sprinkled with a yoghurt sauce and some dill. Indeed a fine health tonic.

Celery

Dr David Lewis of Aston University in England records that when he was a little boy he would watch with fascination while his Granny brewed up her celery tea for her rheumatism. 'It always seemed to work,' he said. 'And when I became a researcher working with a team and laboratory, I couldn't wait to find out celery's active ingredients.'

Dr Lewis' group went to the supermarket and to gardening friends and took as many bunches of celery back to the laboratory as they could. They found that celery extract contains definite anti-inflammatory substances. At least two were found, the most powerful being a sterol of the stigmasterol class.

Granny was right! Only bear in mind if you would like to try this ancient folk remedy for rheumatism and arthritis, that she also intuitively knew that the most potent anti-inflammatory part of the celery lies in the leaves and in the seeds. Celery seed tea also has a strong folk reputation as an aphrodisiac!

Celery seed is readily available from most health food shops. (Don't ever use gardening seeds. They have been sprayed with insecticide and are highly toxic.) You brew up celery seed tea by allowing half a teaspoon of seeds to one cup of boiling water. Let stand for about seven minutes, strain and drink.

The ancient Greeks, who were wonderful observers of the plants that heal, rationed celery when supplies were short. First in line came the athletes in training, next, pregnant women, after that, the needy, and if there was any celery left over, the general population got their share.

Indeed, throughout Europe, herbalists think so highly of celery's tonic powers and ability to sweep toxins from the system, that they advise a 'celery cure' four times a year at the change of the seasons.

Lettuce

Think of salads and a vision of the familiar green lettuce appears, either deliciously crisp and crunchy or sadly limp, resting under slices of tomatoes and cucumbers. Yet what we see as a standard, even boring salad green is viewed with enormous respect as a natural tranquilliser and sedative.

Lettuce contains a white milky latex called lactucarium. This is dried and used medically in pastels or lozenges as a sedative for irritating coughs.

In France, Eau De Laitue is distilled from lettuce and prescribed by doctors as a mild sedative for jangled nerves. The French too have developed ways of concentrating lettuces' power in their time-honoured lettuce teas and soups.

Carrot

Carrot has a normalising effect on the entire system because it is the richest source of Vitamin A which the body can quickly assimilate. It also contains an excellent supply of Vitamins B, C, D, E, G and K and it helps promote the appetite as well as assisting digestion.

The ancient Greeks called the carrot 'philon' because they used to eat the root as an aphrodisiac before making love. The modern name comes from the Latin carota, which means to burn, probably because of the reddish colour of the root.

Carrots belong to the same family as celery, parsnips, caraway and dill and grow in all sizes and shapes.

As an energy source carrot juice is unparalleled for it is

such a good source of minerals that it helps promote cleansing, assists in the building of healthy tissue, skin and teeth and prevents infection in the eyes and mucous membrane.

Some people find the taste too strong alone. It can be mixed successfully with apple or pear juice and with chlorophyll or celery juice. Carrot juice is also exotic in flavour when blended with a touch of cream.

But be careful not to overdo the carrot juice. Taken in very large quantities it can lead to Vitamin A poisoning. No more than 500 ml of carrot juice should be consumed in one day.

Apple
This is a very popular juice at Hopewood because it is an important source of Vitamin C, even though oranges and lemons and tomatoes have a higher Vitamin C content. Apples contain lots of minerals as well as pectin, malic acid and tannic acid which are wonderful purifiers of the digestive tract.

As a blood purifier and general tonic, there is nothing better than apple juice which also contains Vitamins B1, B2, niacin, carotene, Vitamin B6, biotin and folic acid, as well as potassium and phosphorus.

An excellent drink for flushing the kidneys and controlling digestive upset, apple juice must be served freshly squeezed because it cannot be stored, even in a refrigerator, as it oxidises, quickly turning brown.

Pawpaw
This is a treasure house of proteolytic enzymes which are chemicals that assist the digestion of foods. Papain is the most important of these and it is extracted from the pawpaw and then dried into powder form for use as a digestive aid.

The juice taken regularly can regulate digestion and help with the assimilation of food. It also contains fibrin which is a very rare thing for a plant to produce, as it is usually only found in animals and in man. In humans it is part of the blood clotting process.

Pawpaw contains high levels of Vitamin A and C, very little fat and a bit of protein. It makes a wonderful therapeutic digestive drink and can be easily combined with pineapple juice, another excellent beverage with easy digestive properties.

Pineapple
This contains the protein digestant bromelain and is comparable in potency with Pepsin and Papain, for it can digest 1000 times its weight in protein. It is available on a year round basis, so fresh pineapple is a great way to have fresh Vitamin C during winter when other fresh fruits are hard to get.

The juice helps relieve sore throats and bronchitis and will help dissolve mucous formations, while assisting the function of the kidneys.

Pineapples also contain high levels of Vitamins A, B-complex and C, plus the minerals iodine, magnesium, manganese, potassium, calcium, phosphorus, iron and sulfur. As well they provide citric and malic acids.

But don't think you are getting all the nutrients by drinking pineapple juice from a can. Even the canned juice with no added sugar, has lost two-thirds of its nutritional value and all its enzymes (remember enzymes are destroyed by heat during the canning process).

Chlorophyll
This is extracted from the green leaves of plants and makes a valuable health drink, especially if it is taken from the tops of root vegetables such as beet leaves, carrot tops,

turnip and parsnip tops. Another great source of chlorophyll is alfalfa leaves. Called a 'green drink', it provides energy renewal and is a wonderful treatment for such conditions as anaemia, artery problems, bad breath and feeling of exhaustion from prolonged tension.

It contains large amounts of the important mineral magnesium and this is particularly good for people with digestive problems and for those who have lost their appetite.

At Hopewood we use chlorophyll as part of our juice programme where possible, for it is a wonderful way of balancing the daily fruit and vegetable juice intake.

15
Food Can Cure

Today many health care workers believe that remaining healthy is not a precarious state. It is the norm, the inevitable product of properly functioning organs and tissues.

Think how healthy you would feel if you were on a permanent, relaxing holiday on a tropical island, or in a quiet mountain hideaway. There'd be no feelings of tension and stress which inevitably builds as we push ourselves beyond our limit, both at work and in our leisure hours.

The body is one big rollercoaster of interrelated actions. Hurried meals, late nights and lacklustre food, invariably take their toll.

The only way to cope with a fast-lane lifestyle is to pay attention to your diet, to your exercise and to the amounts of sleep and rest you give yourself. Learn to cope with stress and make sure you communicate clearly so that others don't misunderstand you. Chances are, you'll be able to retain that 'holiday feeling' throughout the year.

Good health promotes inner calm and contentment and these together encourage feelings of wellbeing and a desire to be active. Instead of wishing you could stay on holiday forever, just adjust your life, the way you did while you were on holiday.

And true health gives positive feedback. You experience feelings of strength and vigour, a sense of wellbeing and distinct pleasure in all your activities. Unconsciously a healthy person can't help but give spontaneous expression to his/her healthy feelings by being relaxed and energetic all at the same time. Which explains why such people will burst out with: 'I feel like I could jump out of my skin.'

Children who are healthy appear to have boundless energy which, when it runs out, is replenished by deep relaxing sleep. Adults give up this childlike state of health because of physical and mental abuse in the form of stress, anxiety, inadequate diet, bad habits like smoking and drinking alcohol, lack of proper sleep and exercise.

But age is *not* the stealer of health. I know because I am pushing forty and I feel like a young man. I've talked to dozens of people older than me, who have regained their feelings of vitality and energy. Most say they feel better and more active than they did when young.

The good news is that natural food and plenty of rest can cure a depleted, de-energised body at any age, causing the spirits to fly. Just as falling in love at any age, can suddenly improve the health and make the world seem like a special place.

For centuries the common view held was that disease was inevitable. Today we know that it's not. If you follow a healthy lifestyle you can strengthen your immune system to withstand biological attacks. Conversely, disease will always flourish if you live in unclean, squalid conditions and allow your body to become frail and unkempt.

Eating well is not the only way to remain consistently healthy. How you think and feel and how you cope with stress, is strongly interlinked with your physical wellbeing. That is why we have to pay attention to both the mind and the body if we wish to achieve and maintain optimum health. It is said that man does not live by bread alone. And today more than ever this is true. Which is why we need to live in a healthy environment, have a satisfying and productive job, economic security, a clean, warm home, suitable mental hobbies, enough self-expression, satisfying companionship, a supportive family life and the freedom to come and go in a co-operative accepting community.

If we learn to balance these elements, we are simply establishing the 'language of health'.

We know that feelings such as sight, sound, taste, smell and emotions deeply affect the functions of the lungs, heart, stomach, intestines, liver, kidneys and the various glands of the body.

Take grief for instance. It can put you off your food, suspend the secretion of the digestive juices and the muscular actions in the stomach. Joy and happiness on the other hand, accelerate all these functions.

For me, the true test of health is to be always *un*conscious of my stomach, my heart, my bowels and any other internal parts of my body. If you do notice them then they are telling you that all is not well within.

But bad diet can definitely kill if we don't pay special attention to what we eat. All through his working years Dr William Hay maintained that too much refined carbohydrates and incompatible food combinations caused degenerative disease of one kind or another. He was supported many years later by T. L. Cleave in his book *The Saccharine Disease* which indicted refined sugary foods. 'They are responsible for such health problems as chronic constipation with its complications such as varicose veins and haemorrhoids, obesity, diabetes, skin diseases, dental decay and periodontal disease, urinary tract infections such as cystitis, and coronary disease.'

Of course Cleave noted that 'it takes time for the consumption of refined carbohydrates to produce these diseases, most of which have differing incubating periods.

In the case of diabetes, it may not become apparent for twenty years, while coronary heart disease, which was rare in the 1920s, may take thirty years.'

Let's examine some of the diseases which can be directly related to diet and which can be improved by proper FOOD COMBINING.

Constipation

Dr Hay, 50 years ago, believed constipation was a very serious threat to good health. Present-day medical findings have found that constipation is a contributing factor to the high rate of bowel cancer in rich, western nations.

A study paper by Dr Lionel J. Picton in England before the Second World War drew attention to a laboratory experiment on dogs carried out by the famous Russian scientist, Ivan Pavlov. The experiment threw up the following: minced beef fed to a dog is digested in about four hours; starch by itself passes through the dog's stomach in a much shorter time — about one and a half hours; white bread passes more slowly than brown bread; vegetables with bread or meat did not slow up either digestive process. Pavlov then noted that when meat was mixed with starchy bread, there was a protracted delay in the digestion tract.

Picton believed the Pavlov experiments provided outstanding proof that starch and protein are incompatible foods and contribute to ill health over a long term.

Indigestion

Indigestion shows itself in the form of upper abdominal pain, heartburn and sometimes acid regurgitation. We have all experienced these separately, or together, at one time or another. It may surprise you to know that these symptoms are most frequently caused by bad food combinations, rather than overeating and can be cured quickly by proper FOOD COMBINING.

The famous British actor, Sir John Mills, was invalided out of the army 40 years ago with a man-sized duodenal ulcer. He writes, in the introduction to Doris Grant's book *Food Combining for Health*, that he was given the usual ulcer-sufferer's diet of rice puddings, mashed potatoes and so on. After three months he still felt terrible. His sister suggested to his wife Mary Haley Bell that she put him on a FOOD COMBINING diet. Within six weeks he was able to start work on a film and has been remarkably healthy ever since.

Sir John is now an octagenarian, full of vitality and energy and still a working actor. He attributes both his and his wife's good health entirely to a simple FOOD COMBINING programme and to the balance of alkaline to acid foods that he eats.

Naturopath Harry Benjamin also believes that correctly combining meals is the way to avoid digestive troubles. In his book *Your Diet in Health and Disease* he recommends cutting out bread and potatoes with every protein meal.

Antacids, the most common cure for indigestion, are not a harmless panacaea. Most doctors today say they only compound the trouble. There are even recent medical warnings that antacids can use up certain vital vitamins in the body such as potassium. And at Cornell University it was found that bicarbonate of soda and milk caused a form of kidney stones in laboratory animals.

Arthritis
Arthritis continues to baffle the medical profession, but at Hopewood improvements in arthritis sufferers are commonplace.

Lorraine Palmer came to us with inflamed joints in her hips and knees. She found it hard to walk, so had stopped her daily walks, compounding the pain in her legs by inactivity. She suffered severe pain in her right shoulder following a fall twelve months before and this was being kept in check with anti-inflammatory medication.

We found her diet typical of that eaten by older people who live alone. She ate a lot of meat, practically no green vegetables, little fruit and drank sugar-rich milkshakes daily, believing they would keep up the calcium supply to her bones and prevent her from getting osteoporosis.

A week at Hopewood, beginning with a juice fast for three days to get rid of the waste products which were building in her joints, followed by a vegetarian diet of fresh fruit for breakfast, salad and protein for lunch, and steamed vegetables for dinner, left her with reduced pain and the determination to give up her medication and continue improving her condition through diet.

Arthritis has many contributing causes. These include injuries, abuse of the body, allergic reactions, infections, stress-exhausted adrenal glands, too much acid-forming food, and Vitamin D deficiency. The end result, is an imbalance in the body's chemistry.

Too much lactic acid accumulates as a by-product of bad digestion. This results in a depleted reserve of alkaline buffer salts. For this reason our treatment at Hopewood is entirely nutritional and often successful. I have seen remarkable recoveries take place and I have letters testifying to the healing powers of a good balanced diet, adequate sleep and regular gentle exercise. (See Chapter 16 for case histories.)

Fatness

Overweight bodies are far more serious to health than most

people realise. Obesity is closely linked to diabetes, gallstones and coronary artery disease. In America, a survey in 1978 showed that more than 45 million Americans were classified as obese and that obesity among children was reaching epidemic proportions.

Fad diets are still the best-selling books, along with cook books, yet being overweight can be dealt with gently and simply by following FOOD COMBINING principles. There is no need to follow crash weight loss programmes which only serve to put the body into a crisis mentally. By separating incompatible foods into different meals, you can say goodbye to overweight problems in most cases.

When digestion is efficient and there is a proper chemical balance between alkaline and acid-forming foods, your body ceases to store away the poisons.

The best and easiest diet plan, to follow a period of inner cleansing, is FOOD COMBINING. A typical menu could be—breakfast, which is solely fruit or fruit and yoghurt. (For best results make the fruit one type only each day.) Lunch, is a protein lean meat and salad; dinner can be starchy potatoes, or bread, and salad. (Ideally the evening meal should be lighter than the lunchtime meal. That way you have a chance to move around and work off any excess energy generated by the lunchtime meal.)

To make those starches even more nourishing always eat wholegrain bread, cook the potatoes in their skins and flavour them up with such mouth-watering delights as a dab of sour cream or butter and chives.

Just make sure throughout the week that the bulk of your food is alkaline-forming fresh vegetables, salads and fruits. These will promote good bowel activity and help you not only lose weight consistently over a period of weeks, but maintain that slim new you.

Diabetes

The first thing doctors do these days when sufferers are diagnosed is put them onto a strict diet of fresh fruit and vegetables, banning refined fatty foods, cakes, pastries and all sugars. It works wonders in tandem with the medication.

Allergies

These can respond to a simple, basic diet. That's because irritants, whether food, pollens, foreign proteins or whatever are often secondary causes resulting from a weakened immune system.

It may be necessary for some severe allergy sufferers to undergo an intensive cleansing programme first, in order to build their immunity to even a basic functioning level.

What is increasingly obvious is that each of us has the choice to strengthen our bodies, and unburden our immune systems, thus warding off potential allergies. This can be done simply by giving ourselves the best possible diet, by balancing our body chemistry within and by placing no unnecessary stress on our eliminative organs.

It is interesting that recent research is indicating that food additives may contribute to hyperactivity and serious behavioural problems in children and that a healthy natural foods diet may be the best and only way to control allergies, including asthma.

Influenza

The flu or common cold is a disease that has created a flourishing industry in pills, sprays and other symptom suppressants. That's because it was always argued that colds were the result of germs which no one could avoid. Why one person got a severe cold and another not, was ignored.

Today research has found that flu germs can be found in everyone's nose and throat. The reason some people sicken and others don't depends on their individual state of health.

A strong healthy body that is not weighed down by toxic waste will go decades without so much as a cough or sniffle. An unhealthy body, lacking proper nutrients and with poor elimination, will pick up regular colds every year.

Many naturopaths simply see a cold as a way for your body to eliminate a build up of waste products, hence the running nose and cough.

Nature knows how to cure the causes of fever by removing appetite at the beginning of a severe cold. The smart patient is one that speeds the cure further by resting and going on to a fruit or fruit juice diet until the illness has run its course.

Cardio-vascular Disease

One of the biggest threats to health today is heart disease which is actually the end product of long, personal abuse through bad lifestyle habits and diet. By the time the symptoms are noticed, they are deep-rooted and difficult to cure. We can perform by-pass operations to get round the clogged arteries running to the heart, and we can modify our diet and lifestyle to take the stress off a heart that is no longer in good working order, but often it is difficult to undo all the damage that has been done.

Long term abuse takes a permanent toll and this, according to experts, is brought about by saturated fats, cholesterol, hypertension (high blood pressure), refined sugar, emotions, tension, obesity, smoking, excessive consumption of alcohol and lack of effective exercise.

All the above significantly contribute to cardio-vascular

disease and they all indicate an excessive lifestyle which is far from harmonious or moderate. As long as we take little notice of what we eat and how we live, then we all run the risk of ruining our hearts. Positive action to avert heart attacks is similar to that taken for other food-related diseases already discussed.

A natural vegetarian diet, correct food combinations, adequate exercise and stress reduction all help a heart that's distressed and overburdened.

Stress
Research has shown that we all need a certain amount of stress to function well. However, many people suffer from an excess of stress. This comes about because we seek power, recognition and security and this in turn releases unnatural greed and competitiveness. All this requires us to be constantly tense and alert, which takes its toll on the nervous system. The fear of missing an opportunity produces constant demands on the body's vital organs.

The body needs time to relax, it can't remain in an alert state for long, or the muscles grow tired and taut and the mind becomes muddled under the strain of maintaining such a state. Strain also takes its toll on the nerves, bloodstream, lymphatic, digestive and all other systems.

The result is loss of performance when really urgent demands are made, and eventually health problems such as allergies, indigestion, hypertension, muscular spasms, headaches and ultimately respiratory ailments and heart dysfunction or stroke.

Stress is an insidious problem, for most people who suffer from it are unaware of its presence until the body breaks down. Treatment can only be carried out when the person is made aware of the underlying mental condition which has caused the physical problems. Counselling is then coupled with a change in diet, away from foods that adversely affect the nervous system, such as tea, coffee, cola, alcohol, sugar and refined flour, preserved meats, heavy spices and seasonings.

Arteriosclerosis

This means hardening of the arteries, where the arteries become thickened and lose their elasticity. It comes about because of thick deposits of fat and cholesterol and is directly related to poor diet and little or no activity.

The condition is made worse by hypertension (high blood pressure), but inadequate exercise contributes to this condition.

A change in diet can moderate the pain and in time restore reasonable health to those who suffer from this disease.

Other factors which contribute are smoking, alcohol and the use of aluminium, enamel or copper cookware (stainless steel is the only suitable metal, or you can use glass cooking pots).

The ideal diet is lots of fruit juices and fruit, leafy green vegetables, liquid chlorophyll, a tablespoon of lecithin and supplements of Vitamins A, D, and E, as recommended by your practitioner.

This diet should also include little or no red meat or full cream dairy products, because they contain saturated fats and cholesterol. High animal protein foods such as red and white meat, fish, eggs and dairy produce should be limited because they are acid-forming. All salt, processed and refined foods must be avoided at all costs.

16
Case Histories from Hopewood

I thought you might like to read some case histories that we have collected over the years here at the Hopewood Health Centre.

We have been working in the field of FOOD COMBINING and nutritionally based cleansing for more than thirty years and we have seen some remarkable cases of people with various ailments cure themselves through rest, compatible foods, correct digestion, gentle exercise and inner cleansing.

It is this I want to pass on to you to encourage you to start caring for your most precious possession — your body.

Mr Findus
indigestion
'As I was desperate to find a remedy for indigestion (which was waking me up almost every night in the small hours) I decided to try, though without much hope of success, the don't-mix-foods-that-are-incompatible-with-one-another diet. Now I have to confess, the results have been remarkable.

'Within two weeks I had lost six pounds in weight (which had been creeping on me into a middle-aged spread) without feeling the least bit hungry. The rheumatic pains in my hands have improved and neither my wife nor I have had a cold this winter, despite the fact that my office was full of people with colds or 'flu all winter long.

'I am so grateful for being enlightened in more ways than one and for being given the opportunity before it was too late to give myself sounder health through better digestive procedures.'

Ms L. Olsen
hyperglycaemia

'Suffering from hypoglycaemia has made my life a nightmare. As a child I was always suffering from bronchitis and colds and never had much energy. I ate the usual diet of meat, vegetables, processed foods and dairy products — the foods that were supposed to be good for me.

'In my early twenties my health declined greatly. Day in and day out I was plagued by incredible fatigue, inability to concentrate, depression, anxiety, headaches, insomnia, irritability, joint pains, ravenous hunger between meals, negative emotional moods and many more symptoms.

'For nearly eleven years, I battled through trying every fad that came along — high protein diets, small meals six times a day, bulk vitamins — anything anyone suggested. Doctors told me there was nothing wrong with me. Of course I knew they were wrong.

'Even when I eventually found out what was wrong, it didn't help as I found that the naturopaths I consulted didn't really know how to treat it.

'Then I went to Hopewood and, within a few weeks, I learnt all about food, diet and FOOD COMBINING. Within a few months I had more energy than I had ever had in my whole life. My symptoms decreased, I lost weight and emotionally I felt that at last I was getting somewhere.

'I eliminated meat, refined foods, refined sugars and

junk food from my diet. I began to follow FOOD COM-BINING principles and I discovered the cleansing ability of fruits. Initially I went on a fruit juice fast to cleanse and rest my digestive system. Now I regularly have fruit days to lift my energy levels.

'I eat only fruit for breakfast and though I still have a sweet tooth, I don't deprive myself. I treat myself to healthy wholemeal biscuits and cakes occasionally. A natural diet enables me to increase my intake of food and I have discovered that there are so many ways to prepare foods in more interesting ways than just plain meat and two veg. It has really changed my life.'

John Coxhill
overweight and lacking vitality
'I heard about Hopewood from a friend and checked in to give myself a mental lift before starting a new job.

'I was overweight and felt negative about life which didn't seem to be going the way I wanted it. I saw my new job as the beginning of better, more positive years to come. At Hopewood I was put on a vegetarian diet of fruits and salads. In six days I lost 7 lbs and my energy levels rose following several days of inner cleansing.

'At home I made the commitment to myself to continue losing weight and to maintain my new energy levels. I cut down on my social drinking and reduced my meat meals to two a week, replacing flesh foods with more fruit and vegetables than I normally eat.

'My weight loss continued and to my delight I was losing a kilogram a week. My clothes literally started swimming on me and trousers I haven't worn for 10 years suddenly fitted. Overall I went from 97 kilograms to 86 kilograms, which I have maintained despite the fact that I continue to eat a semi-vegetarian diet.

'I've taken up tennis and jogging along the beach, because I now need an outlet for the surplus energy this new way of living has given me.'

And here are some more case histories from guests who have stayed at Hopewood.

Mrs E. M. 59 years
high blood pressure, underactive thyroid gland
Since coming to Hopewood she has changed and improved her lifestyle dramatically. She eats no refined sugar or foods made with sugar. Since practising FOOD COMBINING, she has taken no more Alka-seltzer. She reports improvements in her digestion and has no burping episodes that once plagued her. She now appreciates the flavours of foods in their natural state for the first time.

Mrs C. H. 58 years
migraine sufferer
She chose to switch to a vegetarian food programme after her first stay at Hopewood about a year ago. This change, as well as FOOD COMBINING, leaves Mrs C. H. feeling 'light after meals'. She has more energy, has lost her customary sluggishness, and her migraines have improved markedly.

Mr K. H. 60 years
high cholesterol, high blood pressure, arthritis and headaches
The Hopewood way plus FOOD COMBINING has helped Mr K. H. keep his weight and cholesterol down and his energy up. Mr K. H. also reports an absence of headaches when he 'stays on the path' as he puts it.

Mrs M. F. 38 years
chronic gastro-intestinal problems
She gets a great deal of benefit from the FOOD COMBINING principles. She reports a definite improvement in her digestion, unaccompanied by her usual bloating. Her energy levels are also improved.

Miss P. W. 45 years
chronic and severe dyspepsia, back troubles and exhaustion
FOOD COMBINING has been of great assistance to Miss P., helping her with digestion, losing weight and increasing energy levels.

Miss S. S. 35 years
exhaustion and stress
Came to Hopewood with digestion problems and suffering from stress and exhaustion. A rest, inner cleansing followed by fruit and salads properly combined, raised her energy levels considerably. She now follows FOOD COMBINING principles and has cut out alcohol, coffee and tea and says she is now managing to cope with her stressful job.

Mrs S. G. 32 years
bad digestion and bloating during pregnancy
Improved digestion followed after one week of FOOD COMBINING. She now has less bloating and no pain in the abdominal area and says that FOOD COMBINING helps her control her weight.

17
What is a Healthy Lifestyle?

We can consciously choose health and prolong our active life right through to old age. Or we can take no responsibility for the way we live and subconsciously participate in a slow and painful, premature death. The choice is there for every one of us. All it takes is a commitment to ourselves and a strong desire to live life one hundred per cent.

By this I mean making no compromises when it comes to living in a healthy way.

I'm not a fanatic. I don't mind the occasional beer or glass of wine. But I *choose* not to drink alcohol regularly for my health's sake. I enjoy being active, looking good and feeling well. It's a natural state we can all enjoy, if we feel good about who we are and what we do.

Mental and physical states go hand in hand, so a natural healthy lifestyle goes hand-in-hand with a good mental attitude. It means you shed that mental luggage such as guilt and self hate, and promote an inner patience and compassion with yourself, when you let yourself down — as we all do from time to time.

Love yourself and others will pick up on your energy and respond to you. Be proud of the way you take care of your appearance. A house proud woman knows how much effort it takes to make her home sparkle. It takes less effort to keep your body in 'house proud' condition if you start before you get ill and rundown. Don't fill your stomach with junk foods and cheat on yourself with chocolates and pastries. That is the equivalent of leaving old papers and magazines around the house and expecting them not to be noticed.

A healthy lifestyle is far easier to achieve than climbing mountains. It's a case of making a commitment to yourself and sticking to it.

And it is not as difficult as you may first imagine, because the whole process is self-reinforcing. For example, if you establish a regular exercise programme, you are less inclined to eat rubbish food or consume excessive amounts of alcohol. Your inclination is not to drink liquor and eat unhealthy food, because you prefer it that way. So you see there is no ongoing battle riddled with guilt and thoughts such as 'I shouldn't be doing this or that'.

The process quickly becomes easier with a little perseverance. A daily brisk walking programme may be a drag at first, but once you have gained a little fitness, you actually begin to feel that something special is missing if you skip a few days.

Here are some important pointers to get you into tip top mental and physical condition.

Develop Positive Attitudes
Positive people live positive lives and attract positivity to themselves. Stop blaming others for your problems. Begin to take responsibility for your own life. Consciously say only positive things about yourself and other people. Use affirmations and visualisation to change negative programmes in your sub-conscious mind to positive attitudes.

Gain attention in a positive way. This will help overcome complexes. One way to be noticed is by achievement.

That is why people run faster races, climb higher mountains or breed better roses.

Don't judge others. If you do, you will live in pain and fear that others will judge you in turn. Unfortunately the saying 'As you sow, so shall you reap' is painfully true.

Train people to treat you well. If you are being treated badly, start looking at the messages you are giving out. Stand guard over your mouth. Be aware of what you are saying at all times.

Drink Pure Water

Thirst indicates that we need pure water and nothing else. True thirst also indicates the amount of water that we need.

Avoid drinks which contain the stimulants caffeine, tannin and alcohol, or sugar or chemical additives. Use instead herb teas, cereal coffees, fruit or vegetable juices or mineral water.

Tap water is not pure. Fluoride is toxic and accumulates in the body. Chlorine destroys Vitamin E, harms the bioflora in the stomach and may form carcinogenic compounds. Unintended pollutants in tap water may include pesticides, herbicides, fertilisers and small amounts of toxic metals such as mercury, cadmium and lead, also algae and radioactive residues.

Pure water may be obtained in the following ways — fruit and bulky vegetables are 75 per cent to 90 per cent water, but only if grown organically and in pollution-free areas. Rainwater is pure only well away from cities. Distilled water may be pure, though not always. Boiled water has lost bacteria and chlorine, but not much else. Mineral water contains too many inorganic minerals, such as sodium chloride (common salt). Bottled pure water may be excellent. Or consider buying your own purifier. (But refer back to Chapter 11 for more information on water.)

Self-Healing
Infectious disease is not primarily an attack on the body by some foreign agent. It is a breakdown of our self-healing mechanism. Our bodies' immune system is a defence mechanism against germs which are basically nature's scavengers.

The true cause of disease is an accumulation of toxic waste products and a chemical imbalance in the body resulting from faulty nutrition, incompatible foods, stress, lack of exercise and pollution. Chronic disease and degenerative disease results from suppressing acute disease and continuing to add to the cause over many years.

If organs and other tissues are not destroyed, they have the capacity to heal themselves. The human body, given the right conditions, is a near-perfect, self-healing mechanism.

Healing requires a lot of energy which the body must conserve for the process. Total rest is required. By that I mean physical rest, physiological rest (fasting or juice dieting), mental rest and sensory (eyes, ears, nose) rest.

Mild fever is nearly always a sign of adequate vitality for healing. Don't suppress it, allow it to run its course. In degenerative disease, there is usually no fever and the capacity for healing is difficult to assess.

But remember, vitality can be restored by a healthy lifestyle whatever your age.

Breathe Fresh Air
To obtain abundant energy from our food, we need abundant oxygen. Most people breathe shallowly, which leads to lethargy, acidosis and slow brain function. Faulty posture restricts breathing, so sit and stand up straight, with shoulders back.

Deep-breathing floods the organs and tissues with oxygen and reduces the workload of the heart. Deep breathing is also nature's tranquilliser and anti-stressor. And of course exercise encourages deep breathing.

Always breathe through the nose to cleanse, warm and moisten the air. When deep breathing, inhale and exhale slowly and steadily, taking up to 8 seconds each way. Keep your shoulders back and empty lungs completely. If not exercising, limit deep breaths to 10–15 at a time to avoid hyperventilation.

Regularly through the day, take a few deep breaths and feel the tension drain away.

Sunshine

Direct sunlight on the skin produces Vitamin D and imparts vitality to the entire body. Sick or injured people heal more quickly when exposed briefly to the sun. However, skin damage can occur in 10–12 minutes so limit your exposure and *always* wear sun protection creams or lotions, depending on your skin type. Avoid the hottest sun in the middle of the day. If you cannot sunbathe daily, at least spend some time walking outdoors.

Sunbathe safely in direct sunlight, some of which we need.

As the ozone layer in the upper atmosphere gets thinner, we need to reduce our exposure to direct sunlight.

Listen to your body and don't burn, it means you've overdone it. Don't forget we are talking about *sunbathing* not *sunbaking*.

Physical Activity

Exercise helps prevent disease of the arteries. It increases metabolic rate and is a major factor in losing weight and staying trim and fit. Exercise strengthens the heart muscle and increases the number of capillaries, thus increasing your ability to survive a heart attack should it occur.

It is calming and relaxing and boosts circulation which stimulates the brain, organs and muscles. Sweating clears the skin and helps rid the body of toxins.

Suitable activities include brisk walking, running, swimming, rebounding on a quality mini trampoline, cycling, rowing, tennis, properly designed aerobics, dancing, yoga and Tai Chi.

Nutrition

Eat fresh, in-season fruit and vegetables. They should form at least three-quarters of your total diet. Small quantities of protein-rich foods, dried fruit and starchy food should comprise the balance of your diet.

Try to eat at least one half to three-quarters of your total food intake uncooked.

Aim for a vegetarian diet, or close to it. Meat contains more concentrated toxins than food of plant origin. Meat also is harder on the digestive system. *Combine compatible foods at every meal* for better digestion. Avoid drinking with meals if possible.

Avoid becoming too fanatical about your food. The stress involved in being fanatical can cause more problems than the benefits gained.

Don't overeat and keep your eating between meals to an absolute minimum. Both are important aids to good digestion.

Stress and Relaxation

Stress causes a rise in blood pressure and a release of adrenalin. Organs and muscles overwork and wear out ahead of their time. Stress also devours nerve energy and diverts it away from essential processes, especially digestion and detoxification.

Some stress is essential for motivation and to prevent boredom. Excessive stress can be caused by deadlines, pressure at work, money worries, exams, arguments, anxiety, grief, boredom, competitiveness, workaholism and setting too high a standard for yourself.

Avoid stress by using techniques such as physical activity, yoga, meditation, relaxation techniques, or perhaps take a stress management course.

Develop a positive attitude. Think only about those things that you can do something about. Forget all the rest.

18
Two Week Meal Planner

To help you begin FOOD COMBINING and to guide you in your selection of meals on a daily basis, I have included a 14 day meal planner.

It is vegetarian, but if you prefer to eat meat, then include meat where the protein dishes are listed. At Hopewood, we recommend a vegetarian food programme since these foods are most suited to the human digestive system, especially when they are properly combined.

It appears the real problem for most people is not that they eat meat, but rather that they eat far too much meat. This can lead to an over-consumption of saturated fats and can also cause an acid build up in the body. (Remember Chapter 6 on the Acid/Alkaline Balance?) Over-consumption of meat also adversely affects the amount of waste products we are exposed to, because the waste products are more concentrated in meat than in foods of plant origin.

If you are contemplating cutting down your consumption of meat or switching to a vegetarian diet, then make the transition slowly. Your body is used to your food habits, even if these foods are not kind to your health. It will take a little while to adjust to the change and you must, and I stress MUST, include vegetarian sources of protein if you delete animal protein from your diet. Study Chapter 19 which lists natural foods and make sure you include a variety of different sources of vegetarian protein.

Finally, I have marked the meals as either starch or protein, so that you can begin to balance your daily food intake. As I pointed out in Chapter 6 it is vital to good health, that you begin eating predominantly alkaline-forming foods by emphasising the fresh fruits and vegetables. They must outweigh your intake of protein and carbohydrate-rich foods. In fact the fruits and vegetables should make up about three-quarters of your food programme. Your dinner for example, should be made up of salad or vegetables (three-quarters) and concentrated food (only one-quarter).

Recipes for meals included in this meal planner are given in the next chapter, along with many more.

(Week 1)

	Breakfast	Lunch	Dinner
	each day on rising: lemon juice with hot or cold water or grapefruit juice (if in season) or apple juice		
MONDAY	blended breakfast — oranges, apples, strawberries and sunflower seeds, pureed in blender	wholemeal bread roll with alfalfa sprouts, lettuce, carrot, avocado, beetroot, celery and carrot sticks healthy cookie such as muesli cookie (STARCH MEAL)	salad — lettuce, spinach, celery, tomato, carrot bean bake* (PROTEIN MEAL)
TUESDAY	½ pawpaw filled with green apple, orange, and yoghurt, or as fruit salad topped with yoghurt	lunch box salad with block cheese cubes hard-boiled egg (PROTEIN MEAL)	steamed vegetables — broccoli, cauliflower, zucchini, beetroot, spinach; or salad and baked potato topped with sweet corn, onion, capsicum, mushrooms (topping nicer if cooked) (STARCH MEAL)

TWO WEEK MEAL PLANNER

	Breakfast	Lunch	Dinner
WEDNESDAY	bowl of cherries (in season) or one type of melon—large bowl	tropical fruit salad—pawpaw, orange, pineapple, strawberry and passionfruit, nuts of choice (preferably raw, unsalted). Remember peanuts are legumes, not nuts (PROTEIN MEAL)	vegetable salad (no tomato) Armenian rice* (STARCH MEAL)
THURSDAY	pineapple with grated Brazil nuts	Ry-vita crispbreads with alfalfa sprouts and miso or Marmite or Promite or peanut butter Ry-vita with peanut butter, dates and alfalfa sprouts or chopped lettuce (STARCH MEAL)	green salad apple celery and raisin salad vegetable crumble* (PROTEIN MEAL)
FRIDAY	apricots or other stone fruit when in season, or diced apple, pear and pawpaw	salad sandwich lunch box salad slice wholesome cake (STARCH MEAL)	steamed vegetables or salad sesame stuffed mushrooms* cashew nut loaf* (PROTEIN MEAL)

(Week 1 cont.)

	Breakfast	**Lunch**	**Dinner**
SATURDAY	yoghurt sundae — pears, raisins or strawberries and yoghurt	cosmopolitan fruit salad* — pawpaw, apple, stone fruit nut cream* (PROTEIN MEAL)	hot pasta and broccoli salad with a side serve of garden salad vegetables (STARCH MEAL)
SUNDAY	fresh fruit — apples or stone fruit rice muesli — rolled rice flakes, shredded coconut, sultanas and apple juice	open salad sandwich on rye or wholemeal bread potato salad* with avocado dressing* (available in health food shops) (STARCH MEAL)	vegetable salad bean bake* (PROTEIN MEAL)

* recipes to be found in next chapter.

TWO WEEK MEAL PLANNER 125

(Week 2)

	Breakfast	Lunch	Dinner
MONDAY	pawpaw, prunes and nut cream	baked potato and pumpkin, corn and broccoli bake*, plus green salad (STARCH MEAL)	fruit platter of pineapple, pear, apple, passionfruit, kiwi fruit, plus strawberry fruit cream cheese (PROTEIN MEAL)
TUESDAY	muesli (riceflakes, coconut, dried fruit, diced fresh fruit soaked in apple juice chopped sweet or sub-acid fruit or see Hopewood muesli recipe	sesame seed bake* sesame stuffed mushrooms*, hard boiled eggs, green salad (PROTEIN MEAL)	savoury corn and sprouts* with salad veges in season (No tomato) bread, butter, honey, apple (STARCH MEAL)
WEDNESDAY	whole mixed acid fruit plus sunflower seeds	eggplant and mushroom pasta casserole* or savoury rice* and green salad, sweet fruit (STARCH MEAL)	Waldorf salad* with coconut, sultanas and nuts prune cream cheese dessert (PROTEIN MEAL)
THURSDAY	pears, pawpaw, natural yoghurt	cashew nut roast*, or broccoli pie*, grated cheese coleslaw salad (PROTEIN MEAL)	steamed vegetables, and savoury rice*, stuffed capsicum with peanut butter sauce (STARCH MEAL)

(Week 2 cont.)

	Breakfast	Lunch	Dinner
FRIDAY	grated green apple, pawpaw diced, sunflower seeds	barley casserole*, baked sweet potato, fresh green salad (STARCH MEAL)	vegetable hot pot* with snow peas, tomato, onion, cucumber carrot salad plus cottage cheese (PROTEIN MEAL)
SATURDAY	3 whole mixed fruits	nut loaf* and tahini stuffed mushrooms* hard boiled eggs plus mixed salad (PROTEIN MEAL)	sweet fruit platter of pawpaw, ripe sugar banana, banana, figs, dates, mango, sweet grapes (in season) also bread, spreads and apple (STARCH MEAL)
SUNDAY	pineapple, prunes, sunflower seeds	mixed lentil pie*, also several salad varieties (STARCH MEAL)	4 steamed veges, garnished with tomato, mushroom, parsley berry fruit cream cheese dessert (PROTEIN MEAL)

* recipes to be found in next chapter.

19
Recipes for Food Combining

The following recipes will help you to enjoy eating while following the general rules of FOOD COMBINING. The recipes come from a wide variety of sources. Some tend to be fairly simple and those accustomed to highly seasoned food may find them a little bland at first until their taste buds adjust. For this reason other recipes have been included to help with the transition. Some of these 'transitional' recipes may bend the rules a little or may have flavour enhancers or foods that are not strongly recommended for complete ease of digestion. In none of them, however, are there significant quantities of foods that are incompatible.

You may view this as a learning experience and take responsibility for your own health. You can choose for yourself what level of adjustment you want to make and what foods suit you. Whatever eating programme you choose, I know you will discover improved energy levels, better weight management and an improved sense of well being when you eat more of your meals using the right food combinations.

Main Meals and Accompaniments

Wholegrain Rice and Fresh Vegetables
Rice can be cooked ahead and kept in refrigerator until needed.

2 cups cooked wholegrain rice
1 stalk of crisp celery
½ red pepper
1 cup cooked red kidney beans
2 eschallots
cold pressed oil and mint sauce to taste

Mint Sauce
1 tablespoon chopped fresh mint
1 teaspoon honey
2 tablespoons grape juice
½ cup water

If unable to cook red kidney beans then use from a tin, drain liquid and thoroughly rinse. Chop all vegetables into tiny pieces, add to rice and season with cold pressed oil and mint sauce. Serve in a glass bowl.

To make mint sauce, chop mint, add honey and water and bring to boil slowly. Simmer for a few minutes and leave to cool.

Serves 6 STARCH

Pasta and Broccoli Salad (Hot or Cold)

1½ cups Soyaroni or wholemeal spiral noodles
350 g broccoli flowerettes
1 small red capsicum (sliced)
1 tablespoon chopped fresh parsley

Dressing
1 clove garlic crushed
1½ tablespoons olive oil
1 tablespoon celery juice
1 egg yolk
ground Cayenne pepper

Prepare dressing in advance if possible to allow garlic flavour to permeate. Combine all dressing ingredients and blend at high speed. Egg will give it a creamier dressing.

Cook Soyaroni until soft. Lightly steam broccoli flowerettes and capsicum slices. Toss together pasta, vegetables, dressing and parsley. If a hot dish, cover and warm in oven at 180°C for ½ hour. Garnish with parsley.

Serves 4 STARCH

Savoury Corn and Sprouts

2 cobs corn
1 tablespoon cold-pressed unrefined safflower oil
1 onion, diced
½ teaspoon crushed garlic
1 teaspoon oregano
1 cup mung sprouts
½ cup sliced fresh mint leaves
Shoyu or vegetable salt to taste

Lay corn cob flat on cutting board and cut corn kernels off the cob with lengthwise cuts.

Heat oil in pan and sauté onion, garlic and oregano until onions are clear. Add corn kernels, stir well and cover.

Cook on medium/low heat until corn is tender, then add sprouts, mint and shoyu or salt. Stir well and cook for a minute.

Serves 4 STARCH

Soya Beans

2 cups soya beans
1 onion
1 capsicum
1 cup celery
2 tomatoes

Soak beans overnight and drain. Pressure cook 1 hour, covering beans well with fresh water. Drain, chop vegetables finely and simmer for about 45 minutes to reduce liquid. Then combine the two and simmer for 20 minutes before serving.

Serves 6 PROTEIN

Armenian Rice

300 g long grain brown rice
3 tablespoons oil
1 large onion, finely chopped
1 cinnamon stick
750 ml stock or water
4 tablespoons sultanas
4 tablespoons chopped dried apricots
2 tablespoons currants

Heat oil, fry onion and cinnamon stick over gentle heat until onion is golden. Add rice, stirring for 5 minutes. Add stock and dried fruit. Bring to fast boil, turn heat very low. Cover and cook for at least 30 minutes until liquid is absorbed.
    Serves 6   STARCH

Sesame Patties

90 g sunflower seeds (gristed)
½ cup chopped onion
½ cup chopped tomato
1 egg and tomato juice to bind
90 g sesame seeds (gristed)
½ cup capsicum and chopped parsley
1 tablespoon finely chopped herbs (rosemary, thyme, mint and sage)

Combine seeds and vegetables then flavourings and egg and tomato juice. Make into small patties. Bake at 180°C in lightly oiled pan 25 minutes each side.
    Makes 6 patties   PROTEIN

Vegetable Crumble

6 cups of diced vegetables (onion, mushrooms, tomatoes, capsicum, celery, zucchini, carrots)
1 tablespoon tamari
½ cup almonds, ground
½ cup sesame seeds, ground
½ cup sunflower seeds, ground
1 tablespoon tahini
1 tablespoon oil

Using a little oil, gently sauté onion, then add other vegetables, putting those which take the longest to cook in first. Sauté together a few minutes.

Remove from heat and put into a casserole dish with a sprinkling of tamari. Combine 1 tablespoon tamari, nuts, seeds, oil and tahini and mix well. Sprinkle in a thick layer over the vegetables. Bake in modern oven for 10 minutes.

Serves 4   **PROTEIN**

Cashew Loaf

1 cup crushed cashews
1 cup tomato pulp
2 eggs
½ cup cottage cheese
1 cup chopped celery
1 cup chopped onion
herbs to taste

Place all ingredients in blender and blend until smooth, place in loaf tin and bake in moderate oven for 30–40 minutes. Can be served in slices hot or cold.

Makes 6–8 slices   **PROTEIN**

Cashew Nut Loaf

2 large onions, peeled and diced
2 tablespoons cold-pressed vegetable oil
2 medium tomatoes, washed and diced
¼ teaspoon ground ginger
350 g raw unsalted cashew nut pieces
150 g mild cheddar cheese
½ cup fresh raw wheat germ
1 teaspoon fresh mixed herbs (oregano, basil, cumin etc)
2 large free range eggs

Sauté onions in oil in a frypan until tender. Add tomatoes and ginger. Cover and simmer another 5 minutes.

Using a food processor, grind cashew nuts into a coarse meal. Grate cheese into a large mixing bowl, add cashews, wheatgerm and herbs.

Mix dry ingredients then add the eggs and stir in. Add onion and tomato mixture and stir thoroughly.

Brush cold-pressed vegetable oil around inside of a small baking dish to avoid sticking. Pack mixture into dish, eliminate any air bubbles. Bake at 190°C for 45 minutes, until cooked through and light brown on top, for 45 minutes.

Serves 6   PROTEIN

Potatoes

Scrub well, dry and leave in jackets. Bake in hot oven until able to be pierced with fork (approx. 45 minutes).

STARCH

Bean Bake

1 tablespoon oil
1 onion, chopped
2 cloves garlic, crushed
1 capsicum, chopped
1–2 zucchini, diced
½ eggplant, diced
3 cups soya beans
3–4 tomatoes, chopped
1 tablespoon tamari
250 g tofu, drained, sliced
1 cup grated tasty cheese

Heat oil gently with onion, garlic, eggplant, zucchini and cook over a moderate heat for 2 minutes. Add tomatoes and cook until mix becomes pulpy. Stir in cooked beans and cook for 10 minutes. Add tamari to taste. Place mixture in a lightly oiled casserole dish and top with tofu slices, then grated cheese. Bake at 200°C for 10 minutes until golden brown.
Serves 4   **PROTEIN**

Hazelnut and Cashew Nut Loaf

½ cup cashews
½ cup hazelnuts
1 medium onion (chopped)
1 cup each celery, carrot and tomato (chopped)
1 tablespoon parsley, thyme, marjoram or any herbs
1 egg (beaten)
tomato juice or water to moisten

Grind the nuts, sauté the onion in cold-pressed oil and add to the nuts. Add the herbs and beaten egg, also chopped vegetables. Add liquid to a fairly moist consistency. Place in greased oven dish, top with tomato slices. Bake at 150°C for approximately 45 minutes.

Makes 6–8 slices   PROTEIN

Tempeh with Chinese Cabbage and Chives

2 tablespoons olive oil
250 g tempeh
1 onion, diced
2 sticks celery, sliced
½ teaspoon ground coriander
½ teaspoon ground cumin
⅛ teaspoon tumeric
4 leaves Chinese cabbage, chopped
1 bunch chives, cut 2 cm long
1 bunch chives, cut 2 cm long
2–3 teaspoons toasted sesame oil
1–2 tablespoons lemon juice

Cut tempeh into bite-size pieces. Heat olive oil in pan and fry tempeh on two sides until lightly browned. Drain on absorbent paper. In the same pan, sauté onion, celery and spices until onion is clear. Add water and shoyu and cook covered for five minutes on medium heat. Add tempeh and remaining ingredients and cook until cabbage is crispy soft and tempeh has been heated throughout. Adjust seasonings and serve immediately.

Serves 4   PROTEIN

Red Kidney Beans

2 cups red kidney beans
1 onion, diced (optional)
½ cup tomato juice
1 cup chopped parsley

Soak beans overnight, drain. Pressure cook in water for 1 hour after bringing to full pressure. Drain, allow to cool. Add tomato juice, parsley and onion.
Serves 6   STARCH

Lemon Tahini Soybeans

2 cups dry soybeans
6 cups water
2 tablespoons cold-pressed unrefined safflower oil
1 tablespoon mustard seeds
1 large onion, diced
1 teaspoon crushed garlic
3 teaspoons grated ginger
3 teaspoons ground cumin
3 teaspoons ground coriander
1 teaspoon paprika
½ teaspoon tumeric
4 cups water
15 cm strip kombu
2 tablespoons shoyu
¼ cup lemon juice
⅓ cup tahini
2 tablespoons toasted sesame oil
1 tablespoon kuzu or arrowroot
1 cup cold water

Pick through the chickpeas for stones, wash and soak in 6 cups of water for 8 to 24 hours. Drain and discard soaking water.

Heat safflower oil in saucepan and sauté mustard seeds on high heat until they pop. Turn down heat and add onion, garlic, ginger and remaining spices. Cook till onion is clear. Add soaked chickpeas and 4 cups fresh water. Bring to boil and skim off and discard grey froth that appears. With scissors cut kombu into thin short strips and add. Simmer covered till tender for 30 minutes.

Add shoyu, lemon juice to cooked chickpeas and simmer a further 5 minutes. Mix in tahini and sesame oil. Dissolve kuzu in cold water and stir into stew. Cook on high heat while stirring till kuzu has thickened the cooking liquid to a sauce.

Serves 6 PROTEIN

Spinach Pie

1 bunch raw spinach (chopped and washed)
1 capsicum, chopped
2 eggs
1 cup grated cheese
2 onions, chopped
1 cup cottage cheese
herbs to taste

Place spinach, 1 onion and capsicum into baking dish. Make purée of cottage cheese, eggs and herbs and onion and pour over raw spinach, etc. Cover with grated cheese and bake 30–40 minutes in moderate oven.

Serves 6–8 PROTEIN

Lentil Pie

1 cup brown lentils or lima beans
1 cup onion, chopped
1 cup celery, chopped
1 cup carrot, chopped
3–4 cups water
1 tablespoon mixed herbs
1 tablespoon parsley

Boil lentils in water until soft but not mushy for approximately ½ hour. Add vegetables and cook until soft and thick. Add chopped parsley and herbs. Place in oven dish, cover with mashed potato, dot with unsalted butter and brown under griller or in the oven.
   Serves 6   STARCH

Savoury Rice

2 cups brown rice
4 cups water
2 cups capsicum
1 cup onion
½ cup radish
2 cups celery
½ cup parsley or chives
soy sauce, optional

Bring rice to boil in water and simmer until water has been absorbed (approximately 45 minutes). Chop remaining raw ingredients finely and add to rice and place in warm oven for 5 minutes.
   Serves 8   STARCH

Buckwheat Casserole

1½ cups buckwheat
3 cups boiling water
1 cup chopped onion
1 cup celery, chopped
1 cup sliced mushrooms
mixed herbs
little cold-pressed oil
1 cup green pepper

Add buckwheat to boiling water and simmer for 20 minutes until all water is absorbed and buckwheat is tender. Cover and stand on stove until fluffy (about 20 minutes). Sauté vegetables and herbs for 2–3 minutes in cold pressed oil, add buckwheat and place in oven for 20 minutes to heat through.
Serves 4   **STARCH**

Avocado Supreme

2 ripe avocadoes
juice of 1 lemon
4 chopped shallots
½ cup chopped parsley
1 cup ground cashews
⅓ cup sour cream

Mash avocadoes; add lemon juice immediately. Add other ingredients and mix well. Place in serving dish and bake for 15–20 minutes in moderate oven—not to cook but to heat through. Serve with green salad and steamed green beans or broccoli.
Serves 4   **PROTEIN**

Sesame Stuffed Mushrooms

12 medium mushrooms
2 tablespoons tahini
1 clove garlic (optional)
2 tablespoons chopped raw vegetables (onion, capsicum, celery, tomato, chives, etc)
1 tablespoon chopped parsley
4 tablespoons ground sesame seeds
1 tablespoon tamari
4 tablespoons cottage cheese
dash of lemon juice

Crush garlic and mix together with all other filling ingredients. Remove stem from mushrooms and fill with above mixture. Bake in a hot oven, 200°C for 15–20 minutes. Replace stem on top of filling and return to oven for another 5 minutes.
Serves 4   PROTEIN

Adzuki and Pumpkin Stew

2 cups dry aduki beans
water
15 cm strip kombu
pinch sea salt
2 teaspoons unrefined safflower oil
3 cups sliced onions
2 teaspoons crushed garlic
3 teaspoons grated ginger
6 cups butternut pumpkin, diced into 2 cm cubes
2–3 cups sliced celery
1 tablespoon mugi or genmai miso
½ cup finely sliced shalllots

Sift through beans for stones, wash beans and soak them in 4 cups water for 6 hours or overnight. Drain beans and discard soaking water. Bring to the boil 3¼ cups water, aduki beans and kombu. Remove kombu and slice into thin short strips. Skim off any grey froth. Return kombu to pot. Simmer covered until beans are soft, then salt and cook a few more minutes.

Heat oil in saucepan and sauté onion, garlic and ginger until onions are transparent. Add pumpkin and cook covered for 5 minutes. Mix in celery and vinegar and cook covered for another 5 minutes. Without disturbing the vegetables, lay out beans on top of the vegetables. Make a small hollow in the centre of the bean layer and put miso in. Cover and either simmer on stove or bake in moderate oven until vegetables are tender. Then mix miso through. Adjust seasoning and remove from heat. Garnish each serve with shallots.

Serves 6–8   STARCH

Avocado Delight

3 avocadoes, halved
½ cup wheatgerm
½ cup chopped tomatoes
1 cup grated tasty cheese
few chopped spring onions
2 cloves garlic, crushed
seasoning to taste

Mix last 5 ingredients, keeping 1 tablespoon of cheese back for topping. Fill avocadoes and top with cheese. Dry bake on cooking tray for about 15 minutes at 190°C. Serve with green salad.

Serves 6   PROTEIN

Carrots with Orange Ginger Sauce

2 tablespoons cold-pressed unrefined safflower oil
2 medium onions, sliced
1 tablespoon grated ginger
750 g carrots, cut into batons
finely grated rind of one orange
¼ shoyu
approximately ¼ cup maltose or rice honey
1 tablespoon kuzu (or arrowroot)
water

Heat oil in pan and sauté onions and ginger until onions are clear. Mix through carrots, add orange rind and juice, shoyu, maltose and ½ cup water and simmer, covered until vegetables are tender. Dissolve kuzu in ¾ cup cold water and stir into vegetables. Cook on high heat until kuzu clarifies. Remove from heat.
  Serves 6

Tofu Tahini Simmer

600 g tofu
¼ cup tahini
2 tablespoons shoyu or salt to taste
2 tablespoons lemon juice
2–3 cups water
1 teaspoon grated ginger

Cut tofu into cutlets and lay out in saucepan. Combine remaining ingredients and pour over tofu. Simmer, covered, for 5 minutes.
  Serves 4   **PROTEIN**

Tempeh Casserole

Marinade
¼ cup lemon juice
¼ cup shoyu
¾ cup water

250 g tempeh
¼ cup unrefined safflower oil
1 cup onions, sliced
2 cups carrot matchsticks
1 cup turnip or daikon matchsticks
2 teaspoons minced garlic
½ bunch shallots, cut into 2 cm pieces
1 tablespoon kuzu or arrowroot
1 cup cold water

Combine marinade ingredients. Cut tempeh into bite-sized pieces and marinate in shallow dish for at least 10 minutes, turning over once. Drain tempeh and reserve marinade. Heat 2 tablespoons oil in skillet and fry tempeh on both sides. Add more oil if necessary. Drain on absorbent paper and set aside.

Heat 2 tablespoons oil in saucepan and sauté onions until clear, mix in carrots and then turnip or daikon. Cover and cook for 5 minutes. Add tempeh and marinade and simmer, covered for 15 minutes, stirring carefully a few times. Add garlic and whites of shallots and cook another 5 minutes. Add greens of shallots and cook until they turn bright green.

Dissolve kuzu in cold water. Push vegetables to one side and pour the kuzu slurry into the marinade liquid while you stir. Cook until liquid thickens and mix through vegetables.

Serves 4–6   **PROTEIN**

Vegetable Dahl

2 tablespoons unrefined safflower oil
1½ teaspoons mustard seeds
2 medium onions, sliced 1 cm pieces
2 teaspoons crushed garlic
2 teaspoons grated ginger
1½ teaspoons ground cumin
1½ teaspoons ground coriander
1½ teaspoons tumeric
¼ teaspoon ground fennel
¼ teaspoon kibbled pepper
¼ teaspoon paprika
¼ teaspoon ground cardamon
2 carrots, sliced into 1 cm pieces
1 cup cubed butternut pumpkin
2 cups yellow split peas
1 bay leaf
6 cups water
15 cm strip kombu seaweed
2 cobs corn
¼ teaspoon sea salt
1 tablespoon shoyu
1 cup green peas
½ red capsicum, chopped (optional)
¼ cup chopped shallots

Heat oil in pan and sauté mustard seeds on high heat until they pop. Turn heat down and cook onions, garlic, ginger and spices until onions are transparent. Mix through carrots and butternut.

Pick through split peas for stones, wash and drain. Add split peas, water, bay leaf and kombu to vegetables — bring to the boil. Skim off and discard any grey froth that forms

after the boil. Remove kombu, slice thinly, and return to pot. Cook covered for 20 minutes. Cut corn kernels off cob and add. When split peas are tender, add salt, shoyu, peas and capsicum and cook for 5 minutes. Adjust seasonings if necessary. Serve garnished with shallots.
Serves 6 STARCH

Rainbow Trout Baked with Lemon

2 rainbow trout
2 teaspoons chopped garlic
½ cup chopped parsley
juice of 2 lemons
¼ cup water

Wash trout and lay flat in baking dish. Stuff with garlic and parsley. Pour lemon juice and water over fish, cover and bake at 190°C for 40–50 minutes, turning fish after 25 minutes.
Serves 4 PROTEIN

Marinated Fish

250 g redfish fillets
3 teaspoons lemon juice
2 tablespoons shoyu
¼ cup water

Combine all ingredients in flat dish and marinate for at least 10 minutes. Lay out in a frypan and cook for 3 minutes on each side with the lid on the pan.
Serves 4 PROTEIN

Steamed Vegetable Sauce

1 can tomato juice
2 teaspoons Promite
1 teaspoon kelp powder
1 cup water
large glass jug of vegetable stock
1 cup wholemeal flour
1 teaspoon Jensens broth

In a boiler cook together juice, stock, Promite, kelp and broth. Bring to the boil and simmer 5 minutes, stirring constantly. Remove from stove.

Mix flour into paste with 1 cup of cold water. Return boiler to stove and add flour mixture slowly. Simmer and stir until thickened. Serve in jugs.

Serves 30   NOT SUITABLE STARCHY VEGETABLES

Bean Shoots

600 g bean shoots
2 tablespoons unrefined safflower oil
1½ cups sliced onions
1 teaspoon crushed garlic
1 teaspoon dark sesame oil
1 teaspoon grated ginger
3 tablespoons shoyu
2 tablespoons brown rice vinegar

Place bean shoots into colander and scald with boiling water. Drain. Heat safflower oil in wok and sauté onions, garlic and ginger until onions are clear. Add seasonings and simmer for 2 minutes then switch off. Mix through bean shoots. Serve hot or cold.

Serves 6

Soups

Split Pea Soup

2 cups dry split peas
8 cups water
6 strips kombu
vegetable salt
1 large carrot, sliced
2 medium onions, sliced
1 medium parsnip, sliced
2 stalks celery
miso to taste
2 teaspoons grated ginger
¼ cup finely sliced eschallots

Pick over split peas for stones. Then wash and drain. Bring to boil with water in large saucepan. Skim off and throw away grey residue that formed just after the boil. Add kombu and cook covered for 30 minutes, until peas are soft. Add carrots, onions, parsnips and celery and cook until vegetables are tender. Season and garnish with miso, ginger and eschallots.
Serves 6   STARCH

Potassium Broth

1 cup water
1 sliced unpeeled potato
1 chopped onion
1 grated carrot
1 cabbage leaf or spinach leaf
1 stick celery, chopped

Simmer for 20 minutes, sieve.
Serves 2

Minestrone Soup

water
⅔ cup mixed baby lima beans, kidney beans and boaurlotti beans
⅓ cup unpearled barley
8 strips kombu (15 cm)
1 tablespoon oil
2 onions, sliced
1 teaspoon crushed garlic
2 teaspoons oregano
⅓ packet of wholewheat noodles
¼ coarsely chopped parsley
2 large carrots, sliced
250 g button squash, sliced
¼ cup shoyu

Soak kidney beans in water to cover for 6 to 8 hours, then drain and discard soaking water. Bring to a boil 10 cups of water, soaked beans, barley and kombu. Skim off grey froth that appears after boil. Remove kombu, slice into thin short strips and reserve. Simmer beans and barley for 30 minutes.

Heat oil in pan and sauté onions, garlic until clear. Mix in carrots, kombu, squash and add vegetables, shoyu and oregano to soup pot and simmer for 20 minutes.

Break up the noodles into the soup until noodles are done (20 minutes). Adjust seasoning and add water if necessary. Mix parsley into soup just before serving.

Serves 6 **STARCH**

Carrot and Coriander Soup

1 tablespoon unrefined safflower oil
2 medium onions, diced
¼ cup fine ground coriander
2 teaspoons of coriander seeds, freshly ground
1½ kg carrots, scrubbed and chopped
6 cups of water
1⅓ cups wholemeal flour
vegetable salt to taste

Heat oil in soup pot and lightly sauté onion and coriander. Add carrots and 2 cups water, cook covered on low heat until carrots are tender. Add another 4 cups water and purée. Add flour and salt and blend through, then bring to a boil and simmer for 10 minutes.
  Serves 14   **STARCH**

Starters and Salads

Avocado and Ricotta Dip

1 avocado, fully ripe
½ cup (125 g) ricotta cheese
1 teaspoon lemon
½ teaspoon ground cumin

Blend all ingredients thoroughly and chill. Garnish with paprika and/or fresh parsley. Serve with fresh vegetable crudites, e.g. carrot or celery sticks, cauliflower flowerettes, or rice crackers.
  Serves 4   **PROTEIN**

Sprouted Grains

Soak 1½ tablespoons of seeds overnight. After soaking, rinse well and drain through sieve or gauze over top of jar or basin.

Rinse at least twice daily, three times if possible, draining well. Sprouts are ready in about three days in summer, 5–7 days in winter. Leave away from direct sun to sprout and place on window sill in direct sunlight for chlorophyll to form.

Wheat sprouts are best eaten one centimetre long; lentil sprouts mould quickly (use them up to three centimetres long). Sunflower sprouts are best one centimetre long. When sprouts are ready put them in a jar in the fridge if you wish to keep some for a few days. They are mainly added to salads, or a side dish but can be used for patties, blended to a purée or as a base for soups or a garnish.

NEUTRAL

Waldorf Salad

½ cup walnuts, chopped
1 stick celery, chopped
1 green (i.e. Granny Smith) apple, diced
yoghurt or mayonnaise to bind

Mix all ingredients then add binding. Serve on lettuce and garnish with fruit such as apple, pear, pawpaw. Top with a few prunes.

Serves 1 PROTEIN

Corn Salad

90 g whole kernel corn
30 g parsley
small amount mayonnaise to bind

Toss together. Serve on lettuce, surrounded by cucumber slices and capsicum. Garnish with any of the following: red apple, avocado, banana, pawpaw or dates.
   Serves 1   **STARCH**

Potato Salad

3 cups steamed potato
½ cup chopped celery
½ cup grated carrots
¼ cup chopped chives
Mixed fresh herbs chopped finely

Place all ingredients in a salad bowl and mix together with one of the following dressings.

STARCH

Cauliflower Salad

1 small finely chopped raw cauliflower
1 tablespoon finely chopped mint or chives
1 tablespoon mayonnaise
dash of lemon juice

Mix all ingredients together.
   Serves 6

Coleslaw Salad

½ sliced green cabbage
¼ sliced red cabbage
1 diced capsicum
equal soya mayonnaise and apple juice to taste
1 cup mung beans (optional)
1 cup grated carrot (optional)

Mix all ingredients together.
Serves 6

Carrot Salad

2 large grated carrots
2 tablespoons shredded coconut
2 tablespoons currants or sultanas
1 cup mung beans
juice of 1 orange (optional)

Mix all ingredients together.
Serves 6

Zucchini Salad

3 finely sliced raw zucchini
1 tablespoon chopped mint or chives
mayonnaise
dash of lemon juice

Mix all ingredients together.
Serves 6

Parsnip Salad

3 grated raw parsnips
½ cup finely chopped dates
mayonnaise to taste

Mix all ingredients together.
   Serves 6

Broccoli and Pasta Salad

1½ cups (150 g) pasta
350 g broccoli flowerettes
1 small red capsicum
1 tablespoon chopped fresh parsley

Dressing

1 clove garlic, crushed
½ avocado
1½ tablespoons olive oil
1 egg yolk
1 tablespoon sour cream

Prepare dressing in advance for best flavour. Prick garlic clove and combine with other ingredients—disperse oil and lemon juice. Add egg if a creamier dressing is required.
   Cook the soyaroni until soft—about 15 minutes in boiling water.
   Lightly steam broccoli and capsicum slices. Lightly toss pasta and vegetables, then pour dressing over mixture and allow it to be absorbed. Serve immediately.
   Serves 4   STARCH

Green Leaf Salad

½ head of mignonette lettuce
2–3 green leaf sections of spinach leaves
¼ red capsicum, cut into strips
½ head of butter lettuce
2–3 tops of celery sticks

Dressing

1½ tablespoons olive oil
1 tablespoon lemon juice
1 clove garlic
1 small egg (optional) for creamier dressing
milled black pepper

Wash vegetables and tear leaves into a bowl. Add the strips of capsicum and mixed dressing. Toss.
    Serves 4   ACID DRESSING NOT FOR STARCH

Apple and Celery Crunch

1 green apple
1–2 sticks celery
1 dessertspoon yoghurt
1 teaspoon cream (optional)

Seed the apple, then quarter and cut into fine slices. Slice the celery very finely. Combine the two ingredients and mix the yoghurt and cream then pour over the mixture.
    Serves 2   PROTEIN

Triple C Salad (Carrot, Cauliflower, Coconut)

1½ cups carrot, grated
1½ cups cauliflower flowerettes
½ cup shredded coconut
½ tablespoon lemon juice

Toss ingredients together. Coarsely shredded coconut is better than fine desiccated coconut. Garnish with fresh parsley or chives.
    Serves 4   PROTEIN

Red and Green Coleslaw

1 cup red cabbage, finely shredded
1 cup white cabbage, finely shredded
1 cup celery, diced
1 cup carrot, grated
3 tablespoons dill or parsley
4 shallots, diced

                                                 NEUTRAL

Dressing

1½ tablespoons olive oil
1 tablespoon lemon juice
1 clove crushed garlic
1 small egg
milled black pepper

Blend together the dressing. Combine all the vegetable ingredients and lightly toss. Add amount of dressing to suit.
    Serves 4   PROTEIN

Avocado Salad 1

In crisp lettuce cups serve mixed together:

½ cup chopped avocado
½ cup chopped apple
¼ cup alfalfa sprouts
   Serves 1

Avocado Salad 2

2 apples, chopped or diced
2 stalks celery, diced
1 chopped cucumber
½ cup soaked raisins
1 chopped ripe avocado
   Serves 2

Avocado Salad 3

½ cup chopped celery
½ cup grated carrots
½ cup sunflower sprouts
½ cup red clover sprouts
½ cup shredded spinach or silverbeet
1 cup sliced ripe avocado
½ cup chopped red pepper
   Serves 2

Avocado Salad 4

½ cup chopped tomato
½ cup cucumber, sliced
1 tablespoon olive oil
½ avocado, sliced
pinch of oregano

Set on a bed of lettuce and sunflower sprouts.
  Serves 1

Dressings

Cottage Cheese

½ cup lemon juice
3 or 4 heads of mint
1 cup cottage cheese
3 or 4 slices of onion (optional)

Place lemon juice in blender. Switch on, gradually add cottage cheese, mint, etc. Blend 1 minute.

PROTEIN

Instant Mayonnaise

2 egg yolks
2 tablespoons lemon juice
½ teaspoon mixed herbs
¾ cup cold-pressed oil

Method as for other mayonnaise. Delightful also on steamed or sautéed non-starch vegetables also.

PROTEIN

Peanut Butter

¼ cup lemon juice
¼ cup water
2 tablespoons honey
2 tablespoons raw peanut or cashew butter

Place in blender and blend 1 minute. Alternatively, place 1 tablespoon of raw peanut butter in a wide-mouthed screw top bottle, mix in 1 tablespoon honey and add juice of juicy lemon and 2 tablespoons water. Place top on jar and shake well.

PROTEIN

Pineapple Dressing

½ small pineapple
½ capsicum
2 radishes
½ onion
1 celery stick
1 sprig mint

Chop pineapple into pieces and blend together with other ingredients until thoroughly mixed.

SERVE WITH PROTEIN OR SALAD

Avocado Sauce 1

large ripe avocado
2 cloves garlic
1 teaspoon coconut oil
¼ to ½ cup fresh water
dash kelp

Blend together and serve chilled.
   Makes about 1½ cups

Avocado Sauce 2

1 large ripe avocado
½ cup chopped parsley
2 teaspoons kelp
2 teaspoons tamari

Blend and cool. If too thick add a little water or oil.
   Makes about 1½ cups

Potato Salad Dressing 1

1 ripe avocado
1 egg yolk
1–2 teaspoons cold pressed oil
1 teaspoon salt reduced Tamari

Blend all the ingredients together.

TO GO WITH STARCH

Potato Salad Dressing 2

1 ripe avocado
½ cup celery juice

Blend ingredients together and pour over potato salad.
TO GO WITH STARCH

Desserts

Cosmopolitan Fruit Salad

pawpaw
apple
pear
passionfruit
or
pawpaw
passionfruit
stone fruit
blueberries

Chop all fruit and mix. Use grapes whole. Serve with gristed sunflower seeds or coconut, and/or cottage cheese.
SUB-ACID FRUIT

Cottage Cheese Fruit Plate

Any fruit except bananas, in slices or quarters on a bed of lettuce. Garnish with tomato, celery, parsley, cucumber, prunes or chives. Place 90 g cottage cheese in centre.
  Serves 1   PROTEIN

Tropical Fruit Salad

pawpaw
orange (or mandarin)
pineapple
passionfruit

Chop all ingredients and mix. Serve with gristed sunflower seeds or coconut and/or cottage cheese.
ACID FRUIT

Palm Island Fruit Salad

pawpaw
banana
dates
mango
grapes in season

Dice and mix fruit, use grapes whole, chop dates finely and place on top of serving, cut banana in slices and decorate on top.

SWEET FRUIT

Fruit Syrup

2 cups water
½ cup dates
½ cup raisins

Boil all ingredients together until fruit is soft. Stand overnight. Blend into syrup. Serve in jugs to be poured over rice.
  Serves 10   SWEET FRUIT

Baked Apple

1 green apple
1 tablespoon sultanas
½ teaspoon butter
pinch of cinnamon
water

Core apple, fill with raisins, top with butter and cinnamon. Prick skin around centre of apple to stop it bursting. Cook in 2 centimetres of water in a baking tray at 220°C for 30–35 minutes. Serve cold with nut cream.

PROTEIN

Nut Cream

½ cup cashew pieces
¼ teaspoon vanilla
water

Blend all ingredients together adding water gradually, to blend to the texture of thick cream.
Serves 1

PROTEIN

Baked BBQ Fruit

Apples, pears

Wrap whole in foil and bake or put on barbecue. Serve with yoghurt or tahini cream.

Baked Rice

3 cups rice
2 egg yolks
1 teaspoon vanilla
1 extra ½ glass water
6 cups water
10 dabs butter
1 cup chopped dates

Boil 6 cups of water, add rice slowly and keep boiling until soft (add more water if necessary). Combine together cooked rice, dates, egg yolks and vanilla, stir briskly.

Spread mixture into an oval baking dish. Top with dabs of butter. Add a little of the extra water if the mixture is a little dry. Cook in warm oven 180°C for 15 minutes. Serve cold with fruit syrup.

Serves 10 STARCH

Fresh Cottage Cheese

2 litres goats' milk or cows' milk
¾ cup lemon juice

Have milk at room temperature. Add enough lemon juice to curd nicely. Leave to separate 3–4 hours. Hang in wet cotton bag overnight to drip well. Save whey and add to fruit drinks or soup.

PROTEIN

Apples and Raisins

½ kg apples
1 cup raisins, washed
¾ cup apple juice
1 teaspoon lemon rind
½ teaspoon ginger juice
½ teaspoon vanilla essence
½ teaspoon cinnamon
pinch sea salt

Wash, quarter and core the apples. Cut each quarter into three pieces. Place all ingredients into a saucepan. Cover and bring to the boil and cook on medium low for 5–15 minutes. Serve hot or cold.
Serves 4–6

Armenian Dessert

Halve avocado and remove seed. Soak some dates and raisins then blend with a little honey and warm slightly. Pour over avocadoes and serve immediately.
Serves 2

Drinks

Carrot/Chlorophyll

½ cup carrot juice
¼ cup spinach/celery juice
¼ cup water

Blend.   NEUTRAL

Almond Milk

22 blanched almonds
2 drops of vanilla essence
1 glass water

Blend. Sieve if preferred.   PROTEIN

Vegetable Juices

Great pick-up or pre-dinner cocktail. Dilute juice with ½ iced clean water.

Alternatives:

1 carrot, celery, parsley
2 cucumber, parsley, tomato
3 carrot, celery, apple

Mineral or Soda Water

Add squeeze lemon or lemon slice to mineral or soda water.

Teas

Herbal teas, hot or iced, are ideal for adults and children of all ages. Fruity ones are liked by children, e.g. lemon, blackberry. Camomile is good at bed time.

Parsley and Celery Tea

½ cup chopped parsley
½ cup chopped celery
1 cup water

Blend together and slowly bring to boil. Simmer 1 or 2 minutes only. Sieve.

Munchies

Muesli

1 tablespoon riceflakes
1 tablespoon shredded coconut
1 tablespoon sultanas or raisins (washed)
pinch cinnamon
1½ cups chopped fruit (apple, grapes etc)
¼ cup apple or grape juice

Soak riceflakes in apple or grape juice for at least 1 hour or if possible overnight. Add remainder of ingredients and mix.

SUB-ACID, SWEET FRUITS AND STARCH

Oatmeal Raisin Cookies

3 cups rolled oats
1½ cups wholewheat flour
¼ teaspoon sea salt
1 teaspoon cinnamon
1½ cups unsulphured raisins
¾ cup chopped walnuts
¼ cup cold-pressed safflower oil
2 tablespoons maple syrup (optional)
½ teaspoon finely grated lemon rind
2 cups apple juice or bancha tea

Mix all dry ingredients in a bowl. Whisk wet ingredients, then add to dry ones to make a thick batter. Spoon batter onto oiled baking trays and pat down to form cookie shapes about 5 cm in diameter and 1 cm thick. Bake at 180°C for ½ hour or until golden brown.
   Yields about 30   STARCH

20
Natural Foods
Their Nutritional Value
and Combinations

Our knowledge about food has grown to such an extent that we now know that foods are composed of eight different elements. These are protein, carbohydrates (sugars and starches), fat, minerals, vitamins, fibre and water.

Food can also be classified into categories according to the elements that are present in the greatest quantity, or according to the most significant element in each food.

If, for example, the food contains a large amount of protein, say more than 10 per cent, then it is called a protein food, even though it may also contain high quantities of fat or carbohydrates. Conversely, a food is not usually classified as a fatty food unless it is almost pure fat or oil such as vegetable oil or butter.

Foods are also classified according to their degree of concentration. That is to say 'concentrated' foods which are protein-rich, carbohydrate-rich and fat-rich foods and which are relatively low in water content. The 'bulky' foods are the fruits and vegetables which are relatively low in protein, carbohydrate and fat, but very high in water, an example of which is watermelon.

A third classification which is extremely important from a nutritional point of view, is whether food is acid-forming or alkali-forming in the body. Acid-forming foods as a general rule are protein, carbohydrate and fat-rich foods which increase the acidity of the fluids in the body. The alkali-forming foods include the bulky fruits and vegetables and these increase the alkalinity of the body fluids.

According to researchers who have investigated what constitutes a healthy balanced diet, we must eat 75 per cent to 80 per cent alkali-forming foods. The remaining 20 per cent to 25 per cent must consist of concentrated proteins, carbohydrates and fat-rich food. This balance, they maintain, is necessary to ensure that the body is able to function in a correct acid/alkali balance.

Here is a list of common, everyday foods. Let's start with:

PROTEIN FOODS

The main protein foods are nuts, legumes, some seeds, cheese, eggs and red and white flesh foods. If you are a vegetarian, the sources of protein will be nuts, soya beans, seeds, unprocessed cheese and free-range eggs.

Nuts, soya beans and seeds have outstanding qualities. They contain no cholesterol and their fat is nearly always unsaturated. They have fibre and are free of antibiotics, hormones and vaccines as well as 'fear poisons' believed to form in the animal at the time of slaughter.

These foods do not form uric acid (which leads to arthritic gout), they do not putrify in the intestine and they form far less acid wastes generally than meat.

Nuts

Nuts are a valuable source of protein and contain unusually large amounts of oil. This oil is thought to be a valuable nutrient for people in good health, but where there is a cholesterol or triglyceride problem, then it is suggested that nuts be avoided until the problem has disappeared.

In the shell, nuts are hermetically sealed which helps prevent the oil from going rancid. Their mineral and vitamin content is higher overall than that of meat. Calcium is five to ten times higher and so too is the potassium. Their low sodium content gives them a far superior sodium-to-potassium ratio.

Nuts are equal to, or richer than meat, in B vitamins, because the protein in nuts is easier to digest than that of animal meat. We need less nuts to obtain our protein (about 85 g per day) than we do meat. Nut protein is a well-balanced food, and when eaten as part of a natural healthy diet, incorporating other protein rich vegetarian foods, it provides all the essential amino acids necessary for humans.

Almonds

These are protein rich (almost 20 per cent) and lower in oil than most other nuts (54 per cent). The most nutritious all-round nut because it is rich in calcium, iron, potassium, magnesium, Vitamin B2 and B3.

The brown skin of the kernel contains tannic acid, an irritant which is best avoided by people in poor health. For those who feel healthy, the body should easily cope with the skin. As commercial blanching is done with chemicals, it is best if you soak the almonds at home in boiling water for a couple of minutes.

The almond is one of the best of all the nuts for the vegetarian as it is such a rich protein source. A large vegetable salad and 125 g of nuts, makes a wonderful meal for anyone.

Almonds are best combined with non-starches — vegetables, and acid fruits. They do not combine well with sugars, so avoid almond cakes and biscuits.

Brazil Nuts

Another good nut but not as good as almonds. It comes from brazil and grows in the fertile jungles of the Amazon basin. Its protein content is 14 per cent, oil content 67 per cent, and it is rich in potassium, magnesium, iron, zinc, selenium and Vitamin B1. It is also high in phosphorous, giving it a poor calcium to phosphorous ratio.

Because of its protein content it does not combine with starches. So eat it with non-starchy vegetables and acid fruits.

Cashews

These are reasonably nutritious, with a protein content of 17 per cent and an oil content of 46 per cent, which is the lowest of all the nuts. Their delicious flavour is due to their carbohydrate content of 30 per cent, which is the highest of all the nuts. Cashews contain high potassium, magnesium and iron, but are low in calcium.

The cashew is a relative of the mango and is a most peculiar fruit. The fleshy part above the nut, is called the cashew apple and is used in Brazil as much as the nut. Beverages and wines are made from its soft, juicy, acid pulp. Cashews are best eaten in the unroasted state. They are parched, which dissipates the acid and the shells are then removed so that in the strictest sense the nuts are 'raw' and a good addition to a healthy diet.

As a protein they are best combined with non-starchy vegetables.

Hazelnuts

The lowest of the nuts in protein content (13 per cent), barely rating as a protein food. Oil content is 62 per cent, and it is rich in potassium, magnesium, iron, calcium, with a very favourable calcium to phosphorous ratio.

These are best combined with non-starchy vegetables.

Walnuts
These have a protein content of 15 per cent and an oil content of 64 per cent, and should not be over-used. High in potassium, but low in calcium, there is nothing outstanding to recommend them except they have a delicious flavour when they are fresh. The oil goes rancid easily so always make sure you only eat them when they are crisp and fresh.

Pecan Nuts
A protein content of 9 per cent and a very high oil content of 71 per cent, they are rich in potassium and Vitamin B1.

Macadamia Nuts
Very low in protein (8 per cent), but high oil content (72 per cent) which is largely unsaturated. An expensive, but delicious nut you can use occasionally.

Pistacchio Nuts
A good source of protein equal to the almond at 20 per cent, with an oil content of 54 per cent. Very rich in potassium and iron, but low in calcium with a rather poor calcium to phosphorous ratio.

Pine Nuts
Exceptionally high in proteins (31 per cent) and relatively low in oil (47 per cent), these nuts are high in iron, but very poor in calcium to phosphorous ratio. Small, soft, sweet and delicious. They are best combined in fresh leafy vegetable salads and with meats. Do not use with starchy foods.

Coconut
A useful food which is high in fibre (4 per cent), but not a

good protein source. The fresh coconut contains only 4 per cent protein, while dried it contains 7 per cent. The oil content is 35 per cent and 63 per cent if dried.

In a vegetarian diet, coconut and coconut milk eaten alone and in a fresh state are very good foods.

Legumes

Legumes include dried peas and beans as well as lentils and peanuts. They are rich in starch and also good sources of protein, particularly soybeans. Legumes are lower in oil than nuts and are a good source of minerals, vitamins and fibre.

Unfortunately some of them, particularly soya beans and peanuts, contain a compound called 'trypsin inhibitor' which inhibits the action of the digestive enzyme trypsin which is secreted from the pancreas into the duodenum. To make the protein sufficiently digestible, they need to be either sprouted or cooked.

Soya Beans

The dry, raw beans are the richest protein foods, being 35 per cent protein, with a good balance of amino acids. Oil content is 18 per cent, fibre is high at 5 per cent and they are rich in minerals and vitamins, especially potassium, iron, calcium and the B vitamins.

Soya beans are processed into a number of other food items. There is textured vegetable protein called TVP which is flavoured with vegetable and herb extracts to simulate beef, ham, chicken, etc., also tofu, bean curd, soy sauce, miso and tamari.

Soy sauce is likely to contain caramel and artificial colour and flavour such as MSG so avoid it. Miso and tamari is made by fermenting soya beans, salt and water for up to three years. The solid matter on the bottom of the vat is miso and the liquid is tamari. Some brands are free of additives and are suitable for use in small quantities.

Peanuts

These are very nutritious, and have a protein content of 26 pert cent and an oil content of 48 per cent.

They may be hard to digest. This is overcome by cooking them in an oven or toasting them lightly under the griller. Roasted peanuts, unless dry roasted, are not roasted but fried in oil and should be avoided. The best way to buy peanuts is raw and unsalted from a health food store and dry roasted at home when you are ready to eat them. Peanut butter is best made from dry roasted peanuts that are freshly crushed and eaten as soon as possible. Also available at health food shops.

Chickpeas

Reasonably nutritious with 61 per cent carbohydrate (starch) and low oil 5 per cent. They have high fibre at 5 per cent and require long cooking time.

Lentils

Moderately nutritious with a 61 per cent carbohydrate content, a low fat content (1 per cent). Lentils require little cooking.

Red Kidney Beans

A tasty legume with a 61.9 per cent starch content and an oil content of 2 per cent. They need moderate cooking and are great in salads combined with freshly chopped vegetables and a dressing.

Seeds

The seeds which are protein sources include sunflower seeds, sesame seeds and pepitas (pumpkin seed kernels).

They all contain high levels of protein and oil, but all have a poor calcium to phosphorous ratio. Overall they are quite nutritious.

Sunflower Seeds
These are very nutritious. Their protein content is 24 per cent, carbohydrate content 19 per cent, oil content moderate at 47 per cent, but they are highly polyunsaturated. High in phosphorous and potassium and rich in iron, they contain high B vitamins and high levels of Vitamin E. A very good seed to eat regularly.

Sesame Seeds
These are so small they must be ground up otherwise they can pass through the intestine undigested. Their protein content is 18 per cent, carbohydrate content 17 per cent, oil content 53 per cent, and they are rich in Vitamin B_3. Not so desirable is their fairly high phosphorous level and phytic acid which reduces the availability of minerals such as calcium.

Tahini is simply ground sesame seeds and can be used as a substitute for butter and as a dressing on green salads.

Pepitas (Pumpkin Seed Kernels)
Very high in protein (29 per cent). Oil content (47 per cent) and carbohydrate content (15 per cent) and extremely rich in iron. Unfortunately phosphorous is also extremely high giving it a very bad calcium to phosphorous ratio, so use only occasionally.

FRUIT

Apple
The apple is the world's most popular fruit for it grows in temperate climates and through history has been revered as

the allegorical tree of knowledge. The varieties of apple are so numerous that to classify them would take a textbook. No one will dispute that the apple heads the list of fruits. It is delightful to look at and fresh from the tree, a crisp and exhilarating fruit to eat.

From it comes apple cider which is good so long as it remains sweet. Apple cider vinegar, apple butter, apple jelly, apple sauce and so on are best avoided because of the processing and the additives such as salt, sugar and spices.

Dried applies sliced and dehydrated in ovens have lost some of their food value, but are still good to use during winter when fresh apples are hard to get. They are also useful as substitutes for sweets.

It is alkaline in influence, classed as a sub-acid fruit and is best combined with other sub-acid fruits.

Apricot
These are rarely found in the market at their best because they are prematurely harvested, but when eaten ripe, at their peak, they are delicious and valuable.

Dried apricots are a good food, provided they are sundried. Care must be used in purchasing them, as with most dried fruits, because preservatives such as sulphur-dioxide or hydrogen-peroxide are used in their preservation and to give them a good colour.

To add variety, dried apricots can be softened by soaking them overnight in just enough water. Cooking is unnecessary and destroys their nutritional value.

Best combined with sub-acid and acid fruits only.

Bananas
Delightful, delicious and a staple food for many because of its high food value and easily digestible character. It is a good food for children and convalescents and is clean

because it is protected from contamination by its thick skin.

While the fruit is green it is mostly starch, but as it ripens, the starch is converted into sugar. When the skin is yellow and speckled with little dark spots, it is most delicious and digestible. Dehydrated bananas are now popular and the process makes them similar to dried figs and dates. In the tropics, unripe bananas are also grated and fried and this is used as a flour like other grain flours.

Classed as a sweet fruit, it is best combined with other sweet fruits.

Currants
This was the name given the little Corinth grapes or raisins and was known as such before the common currant was cultivated. A native of Britain and the north of Europe, it is grown in temperate climates and the common varieties are red and white, although there are about 26 varieties used commercially. The red variety is richest in mineral content.

An acid fruit it, combines best with other acid fruits and with sub-acid fruits. Avoid starches and sweet fruits.

Dates
There are over 7000 varieties of the fruit of the palm, but few of us ever see or taste more than half a dozen kinds. The mature date grows from two and a half to ten centimetres in length. As it ripens it passes through various colours. Artificial ripening makes the fruit an even colour.

A sweet fruit it combines with other sweet fruits, sub-acid fruits and non-starchy vegetables.

Figs
A pear-shaped fruit, it is actually a swollen, hollow

receptacle with a small opening opposite the stem, completely lined with tiny flowers which develop into the true fruits, the seeds of the fig. Four figs are used for commercial purposes. These are the black mission which is rich in blood and body building elements, the Adriatic fig which is the most common, the Smyrna which is delicious dried and very rich and sweet in flavour and the Kadota which is considered superior to all other varieties because the tree is strong and a good producer.

Dried figs have no chemical preservatives and are one of the most wholesome, nutritive and economical foods you can have. They can be kept over long periods of time and resist heat and cold very well.

A sweet fruit, it combines with sweet fruit, sub-acid fruit and starchy vegetables.

Grapefruit
This is a member of the citrus family and, like oranges and lemons, has been used for seasoning meats and fish and as a refreshing juice because of its biting taste.

An acid fruit, it combines with other acid fruits and should not be mixed with sweet fruits or starches.

Mango
This is one of the few fruits which were cultivated as far back as four thousand years. Oval in form, the colour varies, but is generally apricot yellow, sometimes overspread with scarlet around the base.

Juicy and rich it is a sub-acid fruit which is best combined with other sub-acid fruits and sweet fruits.

Melons
Large and yellow-green with a rich flavour, the watermelon is the most popular and cultivated all over the world. It is

thirst quenching and juicy with a heavy green rind. Other varieties are the Musk Melon, the Canteloupe and the Honeydew.

All melons are rich in minerals and great to eat during the summer months because they combine both food and drink.

However melons should not be combined with any other food. They are best eaten alone, without the addition of salt or sugar. If eating melons causes you stomach upset, it is probably because they are combined with other foods such as icecream or are eaten at the beginning or end of a heavy meal.

A neutral fruit, do not eat melons within three hours of another meal. Eat watermelons at least half an hour before a meal (as it passes through the digestive system quickly) or 3 hours after a meal so that it is not held up in the stomach while other food is being digested. If this occurs the sugar in the watermelon will ferment and cause digestive problems.

A neutral fruit.

Papaya or Pawpaw
Second in importance only to the banana throughout the tropics, papaya are a good replacement for melon. They look like melons with a smooth skin, yellowish-orange colour and a reddish-orange flesh. The flavour is luscious and sweet and it can bruise easily if roughly handled. Pawpaw is like papaya and is used to make preserves, jellies, sherbets and pickles.

A neutral fruit, it combines well with both sweet and acid fruits.

Peach
Known as a Persian apple it unites the orange and the apple. Eaten ripe, it is delicious and has a full flavour.

Picked unripe it never acquires its proper flavour. Dried peach is also popular but it is submitted to the harmful sulphur-dioxide treatment which destroys its nutritional properties. Eat it dried naturally to gain the best nutrients it has to offer.

A sub-acid fruit it is best combined with sub-acid and sweet fruits.

Strawberry
This is beyond doubt the most important fruit among the small fruits. The berries should be picked as soon as they are ripe, for it keeps the small berries growing. An acid fruit, it combines badly with starch and sweet fruits. Strawberries are an excellent additive to fruit salads made up of acid and sub-acid fruits.

Tomato
Tomato is in fact an acid fruit, although often known as a vegetable.

It is related to the eggplant, pepper and potato and has been grown grafted onto a potato (the tuber is under the ground, the tomato above) and called potomato. Like other vegetables and fruits, which have high acid or citric properties, after digestion it leaves an alkaline ash in the body which is why those who suffer from acidosis should eat fresh acid fruits and vegetables in their diets.

It is best combined with non-starch vegetables and protein. Avoid combining with starches for good digestion.

VEGETABLES
These are any plants, cultivated for their edible parts. They include roots (beets and carrots), tubers (potatoes, artichokes), stems (celery), leaves (lettuce, spinach), flower

buds and heads (French artichoke, cauliflower), fruits (tomatoes), and seeds (peas and sweet corn).

Vegetables can also be defined as any plant used in some culinary way as compared to fruit which is considered by most people to be dessert and not a staple article of the diet.

Vegetables play a vital role in nutrition giving us important minerals and vitamins. A diet composed of proteins and carbohydrates would not be nearly so harmful if balanced with a generous supply of vegetables.

Unfortunately vegetables in the average household are limited to a very few. Salad is thought of as lettuce covered with onions and tomatoes, and vegetables are limited to potatoes, one green vegetable that is in season and canned corn or mushrooms.

While fruits and nuts are the perfect foods for humans, it is almost impossible to obtain a well-rounded supply for perfect nutrition and health. Therefore it is imperative to supplement these with a variety of quality vegetables.

Salads and lightly steamed vegetables should form the major part of every protein and starch/fat meal.

Avocado
This is a neutral food with high oil content, also a rich source of fat soluble vitamins necessary for good health. Great to use as a spread instead of butter, and will combine with anything.

Broccoli
This is a close relation of the cauliflower and can be grown in the home garden. The head of the broccoli is wonderful eaten raw and chopped in salads or lightly cooked for five minutes and served with a little olive oil or unsalted butter.

Don't overcook it, like cabbage and cauliflower it falls apart and loses its nutritional value.

A non-starch vegetable it combines well with other vegetables, starches such as potatoes, and proteins such as meat.

Brussels Sprouts
A close kin of the cabbage, it is a hardy vegetable which grows well in cold climates. These too are good to eat finely chopped and mixed in a fresh salad, or they can be lightly cooked so that they are still crunchy, and served with unsalted butter or an oil dressing. This vegetable may be combined with starches or proteins.

Cauliflower
A favourite with a lot of people, it is a health-giving vegetable which may also be eaten raw or cooked. Like its cousins the broccoli and Brussels sprout, there is no need to cook it long for this completely destroys the delicate and delicious flavour. Leave in the steamer for eight to ten minutes depending whether you are cooking the whole head or just chopped pieces and serve with butter, oil or a grated cheese.

It combines well with starch, protein and other vegetables.

Chicory
This is a perennial and related to the Dandelion and Endive. It has a bitter taste as we discussed in Chapter 6, which is a beneficial addition to everyone's diet. The small green leaves of the chicory can be used in raw salads, or steamed for three to five minutes in the same way you cook spinach.

Combines well with other vegetables, proteins and starch foods.

Cucumber
This is one of the oldest known vegetables. Though it has low food value, it has a high water content and is a great addition to a fresh, raw, green vegetable salad. As it is closely related to the melon family it can cause bloating if your digestive system is weakened from too much incompatible food.

Combines well with other vegetables, starch or protein.

Eggplant
This is a purple vegetable and thus a member of the nightshade group which can cause problems for some people. It has a black juice which is secreted if the plant is cut. It is best to cut egg plant in 1–2 cm thick slices and parboil about one minute then drain on kitchen towelling. This has same effect as adding salt, etc.

A non-starchy vegetable it is neutral and combines with vegetables, starch and protein.

Garlic
This is a herb vegetable, which, if over eaten can adversely affect the digestive system and weaken the organs of elimination. It should be used occasionally to flavour cooked food and it makes an excellent seasoning, crushed in salad dressing.

It combines well with vegetables, proteins or starches.

Leek
The leek belongs to the onion group and is picked when the plant produces a stem a centimetre or more in diameter and from thirty to forty centimetres tall. It has a delicate and tender flavour and is wonderful used in soups and salads. Delicious eaten raw, you can also steam it for five minutes and dress it with unsalted butter or oil. Combines with both proteins or starches and all the vegetables.

Parsley
This vegetable is used almost exclusively for decorative purposes and usually left at the side of the salad plate or when the dip is wiped clean. Which is a pity, for parsley is very rich in minerals and vitamins and deserves to be a regular part of everyone's diet.

Combines well with vegetables, proteins or starch.

Parsnip
They are highly nutritious, but not popular probably because they are not prepared in delicious ways. If steamed rapidly, like the carrot, or baked in a casserole, their flavour is much appreciated. A starchy vegetable that combines well with all other vegetables and starch foods.

Potato
For some people they are an indispensible staple food and are a very filling starchy base when mixed with other fresh vegetables and salads.

Because of their high starch content they should be eaten sparingly unless you are a person who is seeking to put on weight. The correct way to eat them is either baked, or steamed with their skins. Again baking and boiling time should be kept to the minimum to retain their nutritious value.

Does *not* combine with protein or acid fruit. Combines well with other vegetables.

Treat pumpkins in a similar manner.

GRAINS

Barley
A hardy cereal, in Scotland it makes a great porridge and

soup mix. It is also used in many countries such as Tunisia, Algeria and Morocco as bread.

Combines best with vegetables, fats and starch foods.

Buckwheat

A large grain, in Russia it is very popular eaten as cereal with millet and other crushed grains. Can be used in bread making and in savoury pancakes.

Classed as a starch, it combines well with all vegetables and fats.

Buckwheat and millet are the only alkali-forming cereals.

Corn

Corn has been eaten for thousands of years for a fossilised ear of corn was found in ancient Peruvian ruins. A difficult cereal to digest when dried. It is made into corn meal, corn syrup, corn starch, and so on. The best and most nutritional way to eat it is fresh on the cob, plunged into boiling water for three to four minutes or steamed and served with unsalted butter or oil. It is starchy and is best combined with vegetables and other starch foods.

Millet

This is also known as grain sorghum and produces small round seeds resembling corn. There are many varieties of this grain and in some countries, such as Russia and China, it serves as a staple food.

It has a 73 per cent starch content and combines best with vegetables and starch foods. Does not combine well with acid fruit.

Oats

Oats are eaten all over the world and in some places are a staple item in the diet. They are 70 per cent starch and are very rich in minerals, perhaps more so than any other cereal. The best way to eat them is in porridge or bread. Generally-speaking oats are most palatable and digestible when eaten on their own, ie porridge or combined with other cereals, ie mixed grain.

They are best combined with other starch foods. Avoid proteins and acid fruits.

Rice

This is the most extensively cultivated of all grains and the principal food of more than a third of the entire population of the world. In the East, every part of the plant is used. Rice straw is used for paper making, sandals, brooms, hats, etc, while the cereal is extremely nutritious. However, the unpolished or brown rice is the one that contains the most nutrients. Modern methods of refining the cereal as white flour or as polished rice has resulted in such nutrition-based diseases as Beri-beri.

Rice is starch, so it is best combined with starch vegetables. Avoid protein and acid fruit.

Note: All starch foods combine well with *all* vegetables and should be eaten with vegetables as they are a concentrated food.

Index

Main Meals and Accompaniments	128
Soups	147
Starters and Salads	149
Dressings	157
Desserts	160
Drinks	165
Munchies	167

Adzuki and Pumpkin Stew	140
Almond Milk	165
Apple and Celery Crunch	154
Apples and Raisins	164
Armenian Dessert	164
Armenian Rice	131
Avocado Delight	141
Avocado and Ricotta Dip	149
Avocado Sauces	159
Avocado Salads	156-7
Avocado Supreme	139
Baked Apple	162
Baked BBQ Fruit	162
Baked Rice	163
Bean Bake	134
Bean Shoots	146
Broccoli and Pasta Salad	153
Buckwheat Casserole	139
Carrot/Chlorophyl Juice	165
Carrot and Coriander Soup	149
Carrot Salad	152
Carrots with Orange Ginger Sauce	142
Cauliflower Salad	151
Cashew Loaf	132
Cashew Nut Loaf	133
Coleslaw Salad	152
Corn Salad	151
Cosmopolitan Fruit Salad	160
Cottage Cheese Dressing	157
Cottage Cheese Fruit Plate	160
Fresh Cottage Cheese	163
Fruit Syrup	161
Green Leaf Salad	154
Hazelnut & Cashew Nut Loaf	134
Instant Mayonnaise	157
Lemon Tahini Soybeans	136
Lentil Pie	138
Marinated Fish	145
Mineral or Soda Water	165
Minestrone Soup	148
Muesli	166
Nut Cream	162
Oatmeal Raisin Cookies	167

Palm Island Fruit Salad	161
Parsley and Celery Tea	166
Parsnip Salad	153
Pasta and Broccoli Salad	129
Peanut Butter	158
Pineapple Dressing	158
Potassium Broth	147
Potato Salad Dressings	159-60
Potatoes	133
Potato Salad	151
Rainbow Trout Baked with Lemon	145
Red and Green Coleslaw	155
Red Kidney Beans	136
Savoury Corn and Sprouts	130
Savoury Rice	138
Sesame Patties	131
Sesame Stuffed Mushrooms	140
Soya Beans	130
Spinach Pie	137
Split Pea Soup	147
Sprouted Grains	150
Steamed Vegetable Sauce	146
Teas	166
Tempeh Casserole	143
Tempeh with Chinese Cabbage and Chives	135
Tofu Tahini Simmer	142
Triple C Salad (Carrot, Cauliflower, Coconut)	155
Tropical Fruit Salad	161
Vegetable Crumble	132
Vegetable Dahl	144
Vegetable Juices	165
Waldorf Salad	150
Wholegrain Rice and Vegetables	128
Zucchini Salad	152

Bibliography

Pharmacognosy, Trease and Evans, (Bailliere Tindall) 11th edition
Nutrition and Health, Sir Robert McCarrison & H. M. Sinclair, (McCarrison Society, 1962)
Fit for Life, Harvey & Marilyn Diamond, (Angus & Robertson 1986)
Survival into the 21st Century, Victoras Kulvinskas, (Omangod Press 1975)
Macrobiotics, Michio Kushi, (Japan Publications 1977)
New Dimensions in Health, David Phillips, (Angus & Robertson 1988)
Mental and Elemental Nutrients, Dr Carl Pfeiffer, (Keats Publishing Inc 1975)
Raw Vegetable Juices, Dr N. W. Walker (The Berkeley Publishing Group 1970)
Green Barley Essence, Dr Yoshihide Hagiwara, (Keats Publishing Inc 1985)
Food Combining for Health, Doris Grant, (Thorsons 1989)
A Question of Weight, Demis Roussos, (Michel Lafon 1982)
Natural Antibiotic Activity of Lactobacillus Acidophilus, Dr K. M. Shahani, (Cultured Dairy Products Journal 1977)
Bakteriologie insbesondere Bakteriologische, Dr K. B. Lehman, (Allgemeine und spezielle Bakteriologie)
Health via Food, Dr William Howard Hay, (George Harrap & Co 1934) (Out of print but well worth scouring second-hand bookshops for)

horizontal
neighbours apolize